EKG | ECG Interpretation Made Easy:

An Illustrated Study Guide For Students To Easily Learn How To Read & Interpret ECG Strips

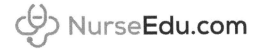

NurseEdu.com

Disclaimer:

Although the author and publisher have made every effort to ensure that the information in this book was correct at press time, the author and publisher do not assume and hereby disclaim any liability to any party for any loss, damage, or disruption caused by errors or omissions, whether such errors or omissions result from negligence, accident, or any other cause.

This book is not intended as a substitute for the medical advice of physicians. The reader should regularly consult a physician in matters relating to their health, and particularly with respect to any symptoms that may require diagnosis or medical attention.

NCLEX®, NCLEX®-RN, and NCLEX®-PN are registered trademarks of the National Council of State Boards of Nursing, Inc. They hold no affiliation with this product.

Some images within this book are either royalty-free images, used under license from their respective copyright holders, or images that are in the public domain.

ISBN: 978-1-952914-09-6

FREE BONUS

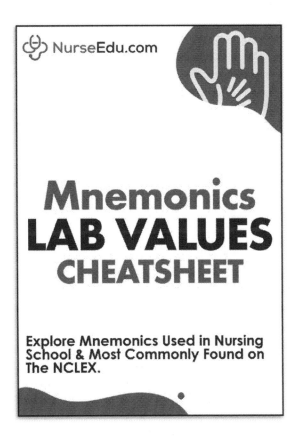

FREE Download – Just Visit:

NurseEdu.com/bonus

TABLE OF CONTENTS

INTRODUCTION

Electrocardiograms (or "ECGs") can seem very daunting when you first try to read them. There are so many squiggles, often visualized in six different "boxes" on the ECG interpretation page. You've been told that those squiggles mean something important about the heart—but what? In this guide, you will understand how ECGs are performed, what they represent about the heart, and what it means to see something you don't think is normal.

Before you get into the hard stuff—the actual interpretation of ECGs, and what to do about what you've read—you'll study the source of the ECG, which is the heart. By reviewing what this important organ looks like and does every moment of your life, you'll see how those ECG lines get generated and what exactly they mean.

Then we'll talk about how the ECG is generated and how you obtain an ECG. What is the difference between a "rhythm strip" and a 12-lead ECG, for example? What is a P wave or a QRS complex? After you learn these, you'll be ready to interpret what you see on an ECG reading.

The rest of the guide gives you the tools to read any ECG and know what it means. We'll cover all sorts of arrhythmias as well as ECG evidence of ischemia and infarction. We'll also talk about what you need to know concerning how drugs and electrolyte abnormalities affect the heart, and what kind of ECG you'll see under such influences.

Did you know? Willem Einthoven was a Dutch physiologist who in the late 1800s first determined that it was possible to gather electrical data from the heart. He created the first electrocardiograph machine in 1901, which weighed 600 pounds. Within a few years, others recognized that the disease they had been calling "Delirium Cordis" was really the sensation of having a cardiac arrhythmia, or what we now call "palpitations." While we call it an ECG now, it was formerly termed an EKG because of the German word for this test, "elektrokardiogramm," and you may still sometimes see the German version in various medical literature to this day.

CHAPTER 1:
ANATOMY AND PHYSIOLOGY OF THE HEART

In this chapter, you will get a clear picture of the anatomy and physiology of the heart. That way, you can know what it means when we say the heart "depolarizes" and understand what the heart's electrical system looks like. From this section, you should learn the details you need to know about how the heart is oxygenated (gets its blood supply) and innervated (gets its nerve supply).

Overview of the Basic Anatomy of the Heart

You probably don't need any convincing to believe that the heart is a vital organ in your body. It is so important that ancient scholars felt it was the "seat of the soul." Its main job, of course, is to pump the four to five liters of blood you have inside your vessels from place to place inside the body. Every cell of the body (except for red blood cells) desperately needs the oxygen blood delivers; without it, some of your cells (such as your brain cells) would die within a few minutes.

If your heart contracts at 75 beats per minute, or "bpm" (the average is 60-100 bpm), this means your heart beats about 108,000 times each day, and more than 39 million times per year. If a person lives for 75 years, their heart will beat over three billion times altogether.

Each time your heart contracts, about 70 milliliters of blood are ejected from it and begin circulation. Your blood vessels add up to a total length of 100,000 miles that must be traversed with each beat.

This makes the average cardiac output 5.25 liters of blood per minute. Over the course of a year, this adds up to 2.6 million gallons of recycled blood (or about 10 million liters). To be that resilient and predictable every minute of your life, your heart needs to be an amazingly built organ.

Your heart is located in your thoracic cavity between the two lungs (commonly known as the "chest"), in what's called the mediastinal space or "mediastinum." A tough structure resembling an orange peel, called the pericardium, physically separates the heart from the rest of the thoracic structures. It largely fills up the space between your spine in the back and the sternum or breastplate in the front. This is what it looks like in place:

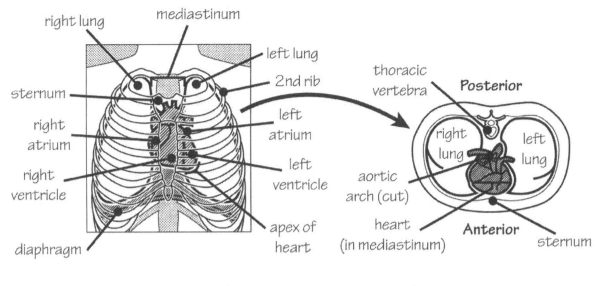

(a) Position of the heart in the thoracic cavity   (b) Cross-sectional view

The heart has an upper and lower border. Surprisingly, the *base* of the heart is at the top of the structure, and the *apex* is at the bottom. The base is where the "great vessels" enter and leave the heart, while the apex is where the bottoms of the ventricles are located. If you think of the heart as a tube of toothpaste, it squeezes first from this part of the heart in an upward direction in order to eject blood out the top of the heart base.

The heart is slightly rotated in the chest, with the right side more anterior than the left. (Remember that the terms "right" and "left" refer to how the person sees their own body, not to how you perceive it standing in front of them). The apex is slightly on the left side of the chest and fits nicely into the cardiac notch of the left lung's inferior lobe. This is basically a depressed area, necessary to make room for the heart.

How big is the heart? It depends on the size of the person. Larger people naturally have a bigger heart. The average size is about 5 inches (12 centimeters) from top to bottom, 2 ½ inches (6 cm) from back to front, and 3 inches (8 cm) from side to side. It weighs about 9 to 10 ounces (250 to 300 grams) in women and about 10 to 12 oz (300 to 350 g) in men. Since athletes work their heart muscles hard, so too are their hearts bigger than average for their size and gender. However, you probably know that "larger" is not always better when it comes to the heart. Enlarged hearts in most people are a bad thing, and often indicate some type of heart failure.

Basic Heart Features

We will go into great detail about the different parts of the heart, but the general sections in a nutshell include:

- **Cardiac Chambers**. There are four chambers in the human heart: two atria (right and left), which largely receive blood, and two ventricles (again right and left), which are the heart's ejecting chambers. The ventricles are larger and have thicker walls than the atria.

- **Circuits**. The heart pumps blood through two separate circuits. The pulmonary circuit, on the right side, takes blood without much oxygen (called "deoxygenated") and sends it to the lungs.

This is where oxygen comes in from your breathing and reoxygenates the blood, sending it back to the heart. The systemic circuit on the left then takes this blood (now called "oxygenated") and sends it to the body's cells, where the oxygen is extracted.

- **Main arteries and veins**. Blood enters and leaves the heart through the "great vessels," including the superior and inferior vena cava, pulmonary trunk, arteries and veins, and the aorta. *All blood exiting the heart leaves through an "artery," and all blood enters the heart through a "vein." The oxygenation status of the vessel does not determine whether a vessel is an artery or a vein.*

- **Membranes and Layers**. The heart is kept in place and prevented from over-expanding by the pericardial layer. This structure itself has two layers, known as the fibrous and serous layers. The fibrous layer is tough and made from inelastic connective tissue, while the serous layer is thin and makes a small amount of fluid surrounding the heart to reduce friction as the heart contracts. The serous layer has an outer parietal layer and an inner visceral layer. This inner visceral layer is really the epicardium, which is the outer layer attached firmly to the heart muscle. The heart wall also has a thick myocardium and an inner endocardium. A cross-section of the heart and pericardium would look like this:

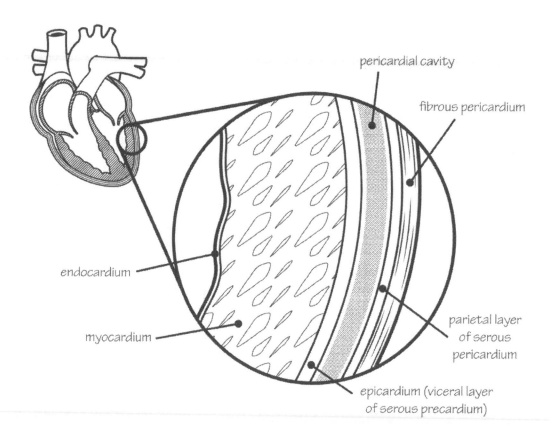

- **Surface features**. The surface of the heart is not smooth. You can see an extension near the top of the heart on either side, called auricles or sometimes atrial appendages because they stick out from the atria. Valleys are also seen on the heart called sulci (each known singularly as a "sulcus"), grooves where the coronary vessels can pass along the heart surface. You'll see that the major one of these is the anterior interventricular sulci, running down the front of the heart, while a similar posterior interventricular sulcus is on the backside. There is also a coronary sulcus that divides the atria and ventricles, as shown:

Heart location and surface structures

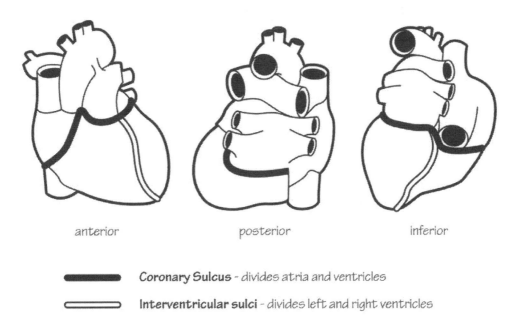

anterior   posterior   inferior

━━━━━ **Coronary Sulcus** - divides atria and ventricles

▭▭▭▭ **Interventricular sulci** - divides left and right ventricles

- **Myocardium**. The myocardium or "muscle layer" of the heart does not have the same thickness all around, but rather is thickest in the left ventricle and thinnest in the atria. It is also not a flat sheet of muscle cells, but is swirled around the ventricles in order to help them pump blood more efficiently. This is what this swirl pattern looks like:

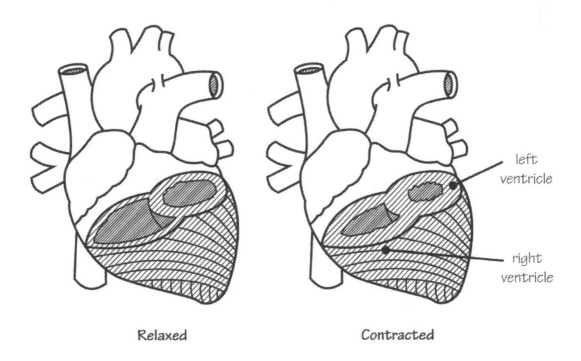

Relaxed   Contracted

- **Inside the heart**. The heart's chambers are separated by walls called septa (the singular form being "septum"). There are several of these, including the interatrial septum (or "between the two atria"). As babies, we each had a hole in this septum called the foramen ovale, that was used in utero to get blood to bypass the shrunken lungs in the womb. This hole should close shortly after birth, but it can take up to six months. Once it does, it leaves behind a depression called the fossa ovalis. A flap near this hole is called the septum primum, and it is this flap that provides the tissue to make the fossa ovalis after birth. This is what the foramen ovale looks like:

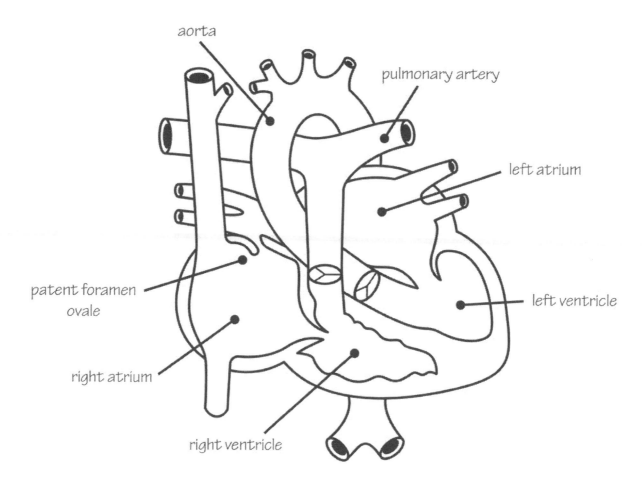

The other two septa in the heart are the atrioventricular and interventricular. The interventricular septum is important because it houses the major electrical pathways of the heart. These septa are reinforced in many ways by the cardiac skeleton, made from dense connective tissue which helps form the heart's overall structure. It is a multi-ringed structure through which several other structures pass. This is what it looks like in the heart:

skeleton of the heart

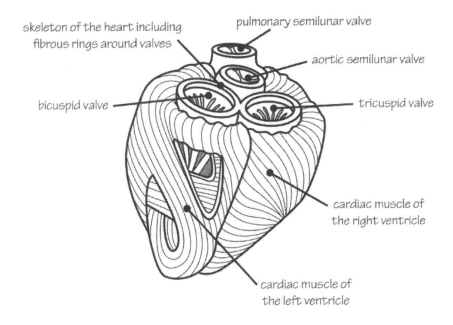

skeleton of the heart including fibrous rings around valves

pulmonary semilunar valve

aortic semilunar valve

bicuspid valve

tricuspid valve

cardiac muscle of the right ventricle

cardiac muscle of the left ventricle

- **Valves**. There are four major valves in the heart. In order of when blood passes through them, they include the tricuspid valve (atrioventricular), the pulmonic valve (semilunar), the mitral valve (another atrioventricular), and the aortic valve (another semilunar). There are no valves entering the heart from the periphery of the body, or from the lungs themselves.

- **Pathways of blood**. Before we get any further, let's look at the path blood takes through the heart, starting at the periphery (the endpoint of the systemic circulation) and ending with the blood reentering systemic circulation. The pathway looks like this:

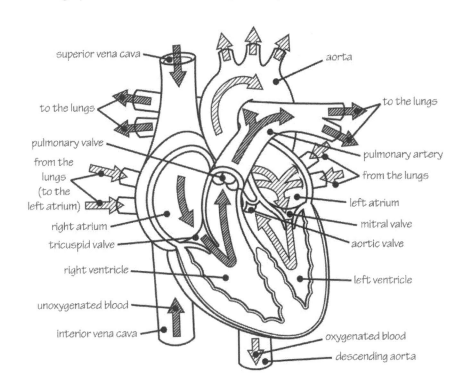

superior vena cava

aorta

to the lungs

to the lungs

pulmonary valve

pulmonary artery

from the lungs (to the left atrium)

from the lungs

right atrium

left atrium

tricuspid valve

mitral valve

right ventricle

aortic valve

left ventricle

unoxygenated blood

interior vena cava

oxygenated blood

descending aorta

Blood enters in a deoxygenated state, represented here by blue arrows. It isn't really blue in real life but more a deep burgundy, even though your veins look blue from the outside. It enters the right atrium through the superior and inferior vena cavae, and then travels through the tricuspid valve and into the right ventricle. Blood is then ejected from this ventricle through the pulmonary or pulmonic valve, entering the lungs through the pulmonary artery. After getting oxygenated in the lungs, the blood enters the left atrium. From there it travels through the mitral valve into the left ventricle. This oxygenated blood (represented by the red arrows) leaves the heart until the next time around, through the aortic valve and into the aorta itself.

Now that you know the basics, we'll delve further into the heart's structures and physiology. Let's start by looking at each heart chamber in more detail, so you know what they look like and what they're for. Then we'll look at other aspects of the heart, including the all-important electrical system, which is essentially what the ECG measures.

Heart Chambers

Now that you know what the major chambers are in the human heart, and how blood flows through them, let's look at each one in turn. They aren't just empty chambers; each has a unique function in the heart itself. We'll look at them in the order of how blood flows through each one.

The Right Atrium

The right atrium is the receptacle for deoxygenated blood. Blood from the upper body enters the right atrium through the superior vena cava, while blood from the lower half of the body enters from the inferior vena cava. This chamber marks the right-sided border of the heart. Its appendage (or "right auricle") is on the front and medial side, its job being to allow for improvement in the right atrium's capacity.

The lower surface of this atrium is a two-part structure, with a ridged separation between the two called the "crista terminalis." This ridge has no purpose other than to mark the two separate aspects of the right atrium, called the sins venarum and the atrium proper. The sinus venarum is in the back part of the inferior atrium, and is the part that first receives the blood from the vena cavae. It comes from an embryonic structure called the sinus venosus. The atrium proper is where the auricular appendage is located. It comes from the primitive atrium of the embryo. Its walls are rough and more muscular than the sinus venarum.

Finally, there is a tiny coronary sinus in the atrial wall, basically a hole, that receives the deoxygenated blood from the coronary veins.

This is the basic structure of the right atrium:

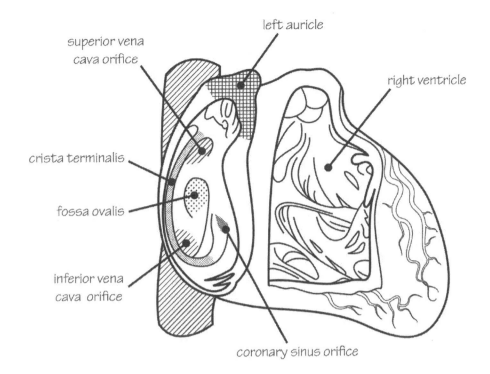

Between the atria is the interatrial septum, a muscular wall region separating the two atria. As mentioned, this is where the fossa ovalis is located. Once the site of the foramen ovale, it closes immediately at the moment of birth.

Did you know? One of the most common heart defects seen at birth is an atrial septal defect. It most commonly happens in the area of the foramen ovale. Most of the time it doesn't lead to symptoms, because the left atrial pressure is greater than the right. It means that blood gets recycled without any deoxygenated blood passing from right to left. However, if the defect is large, it can put extra strain on the right heart, which can cause increased pressure in the lungs and eventually right-sided heart failure.

The Right Ventricle

The right ventricle receives blood from the right atrium through the tricuspid valve. Its job is to pump the blood into the lungs to be oxygenated. The ventricle is shaped like an upside-down triangle and is what you see when looking at the heart surface's front part. There are two ill-defined parts to this chamber, one for inflow and the other outflow. These have a ridge dividing them called the supraventricular crest. The inflow aspect of this chamber is rough and muscular.

The trabeculae carnae form an irregular web- or sponge-like surface on the inside of the chamber wall. These include two features known as ridges and bridges. The ridges are just muscular structures, while the bridges contain some of the most important electrical conduction pathways of the heart.

There are also pillars, which are actually muscles that attach to the tricuspid valves. Their job is to prevent the valve from flopping back or "prolapsing" into the right atrium as it closes. There are three papillary muscles to match the three leaflets of the valve. These are the structures you'll see:

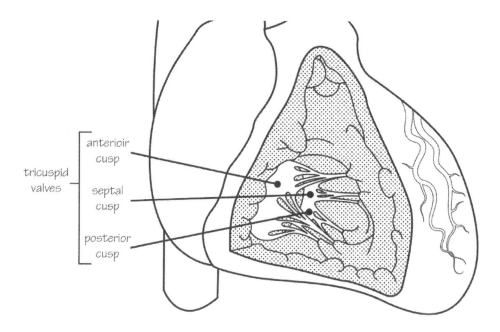

anterioir cusp

tricuspid valves

septal cusp

posterior cusp

The upper outflow part of the right ventricle is called the conus arteriosus. It is smooth-walled and made from an embryonic structure different from the inflow part of the right ventricle.

The interventricular septum is the wall between the two ventricles. It has a membranous portion and a muscular portion. The membranous portion is the smaller of the two, while the muscular layer is thicker by far. This membranous layer is actually part of the fibrous skeleton we've already talked about.

The Left Atrium

The left atrium is another receiving chamber in the heart. It receives oxygenated blood from four pulmonary veins, coming in from the left and right lungs. It is the structure you'll see if you look at the back or posterior border of the heart as a whole. It also has an auricular appendage coming from its upper border, near the pulmonary trunk.

Like other heart chambers, it has two distinct parts of diverse embryological origins. The smooth-walled inflow part is what takes blood from the pulmonary veins, while the outflow part is more anterior. The auricular appendage is located there, and it is lined with its own muscles called the pectinate muscles. The outflow to this chamber is the mitral valve, which leads into the left ventricle.

The Left Ventricle

The left ventricle gets its blood from the left atrium before using its muscular strength to pump blood out to the periphery via the aorta. It is the major structure you'll see when looking at the apex of the heart and along its left border. There are inflow and outflow portions to this chamber, as is true of the right ventricle as well.

The inflow receives the blood first. It has papillary muscles that are attached to cords called the chordae tendinae, which are themselves attached to the two mitral valve leaflets. Ridges represent the trabeculae corneae, just as in the right ventricle. The outflow tract has a smooth lining and is also called the aortic vestibule. In this last part of the heart, the blood flows through before leaving, exiting through the aortic valve to the aorta itself.

Heart Valves

The various valves of the heart help to ensure that blood flow happens in a forward direction at all times. Your heart would be very inefficient if these valves were not there, or if they didn't work well. The blood would go backwards just as much as forwards.

The four valves of the heart are divided into two subtypes, the atrioventricular and the semilunar. The atrioventricular or AV valves include the tricuspid and mitral valves. These are strong connective tissue-based valves between the atria and ventricles. They are both notable for having papillary muscles attached to them, to prevent potential backflow of blood.

The semilunar valves are remembered best if you note that the word "semilunar" means "half-moon." Both of these valves have three leaflets shaped like a half-moon. The two valves of this type include the pulmonic (or "pulmonary") valve and the aortic valve, both outflow valves from the heart itself.

This is what these valves look like in the cardiac skeleton. If you remember that the cardiac skeleton is like a disc with holes in it, you can see that these valves are actually quite close to one another:

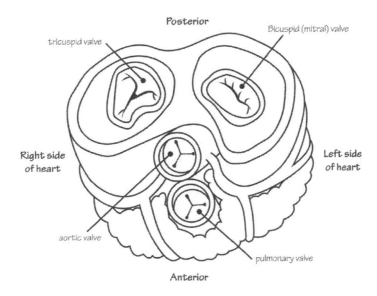

It can be hard to remember which valves are opening and which are closing at any given moment. Essentially, you can think of these processes in two halves: the AV valves both open or close simultaneously, and the same is true of the semilunar valves. This is why most of the time you'll hear a "lub-dub" sound when listening to the heart, and not four separate sounds.

The "lub" comes from both AV valves closing, which makes a sound you can hear. The "dub" comes from the two semilunar valves closing. In some cases, you will hear what's called a "split S1" (lub) or "split S2" (dub), which means you hear the two valves close at slightly different times. Sometimes this is normal and sometimes not.

The two AV valves close when systole, or contraction of the ventricles, start. As this is the time blood is ejected from the heart, you certainly don't want it to go backward here. The two valves are known as:

- **Tricuspid**—the valve between the right atrium and right ventricle. There are three "cusps" or leaflets, called the anterior, posterior, and septal. Each has at least one of the chordae tendinae attached to it. These connective tissue bands are the tendons to the tiny papillary muscles attached to the ventricular wall, so that the valve doesn't prolapse or bend backward during a forceful contraction.

- **Mitral**—the valve between the left atrium and the left ventricle. Unlike the tricuspid valve, it has two leaflets or cusps. The name comes from the shape, which looked like a bishop's mitre to whoever named it. It also has chordae tendinae, but has two papillary muscles instead of the three seen in the tricuspid valve.

These are the valves and the papillary muscles involved with them:

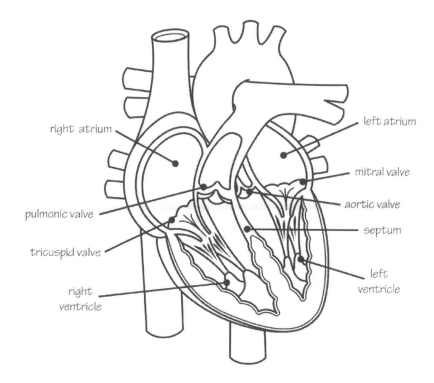

The semilunar valves are known as the pulmonic and aortic, needed to prevent backflow after the blood has exited the heart. The pulmonic valve has three cusps that open out into the pulmonary trunk, while the aortic valve opens out into the aorta. These valves can be leaky (or "regurgitant"), and also narrowed (or "stenotic"), for various reasons.

Did you know? One of the main causes of a narrowed mitral valve or "mitral stenosis" is having rheumatic fever in childhood. Rheumatic fever is a disease that starts with a strep throat infection. Some people will have a strong immune reaction to the bacteria, leading to an inflamed valve. Over the course of several years, the valve gets scarred. This valve will narrow over time, causing mitral valve stenosis years later. It's a good reason to take antibiotics for strep throat.

Both of these semilunar valves are similar, having three leaflets or cusps each. Each forms a tiny cup facing the outflow part of the valve called sinuses. In the aorta, for example, two of the three sinuses have openings for the coronary arteries. Both the left and right coronary arteries come off the aorta directly through sinus openings as shown:

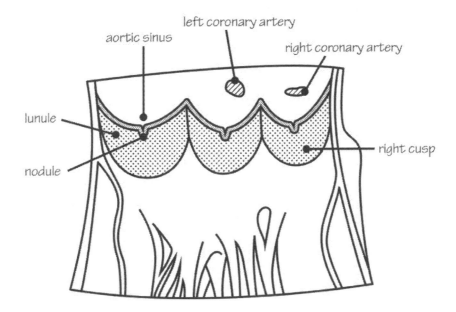

You can imagine why these cusps are helpful. As blood pushes back on them after leaving the heart, the cusps catch the blood and are forced to close as a result.

Heart Wall Structure

The heart wall has three known layers, each of which has a specific function. From the inside to the outside, you'll find the endocardium, myocardium, and epicardium. Let's look more closely at each.

The endocardium is the layer on the inside of the heart wall, lining the wall itself as well as the valves. It is made from connective tissue with an overlying layer of epithelium, very similar to the layer that lines each of the blood vessels. You might not think it is essential, but it helps during development, and afterwards helps regulate the way the heart contracts. This is the endocardium and other cardiac wall layers:

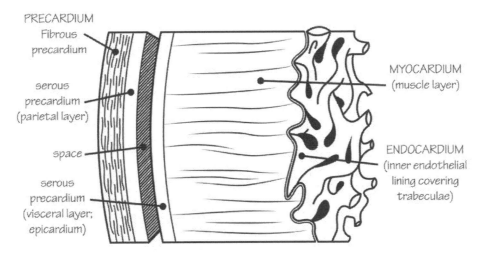

Section of the heart wall showing the components
of the outer precardium (heart sac),
muscle layer (myocardium), and inner lining (endocardium).

There is a thin layer beneath the endocardium itself called the subendocardial layer. It is essentially an attachment point for the endocardium to connect to the heart's myocardium or muscle layer. You'll see later that some of the main conducting nerve fibers in the heart travel in this sublayer. This means that damage to this particular layer can affect the electrical activity in the heart.

The myocardium is very thick with involuntary muscle fibers specific to the heart, called "cardiac muscle" fibers. Interestingly, they are linked together through connections called intercalated disks, even though they are small individually. These are necessary for the cells to communicate with one another rapidly, so the cells can act in a synchronized way.

With the heart muscle especially, you wouldn't want these cells to go rogue and do their own thing. This would lead to chaos and an inability for the heart to work as a unified unit. This is why the heart muscle is referred to as a "syncytium" (even though it really isn't one). A true syncytium is a group of cells that have actually fused together. The myocardium isn't made from fused cells, but they communicate easily with one another because of the intercalated discs, and so are a "functional" syncytium. This is what they look like:

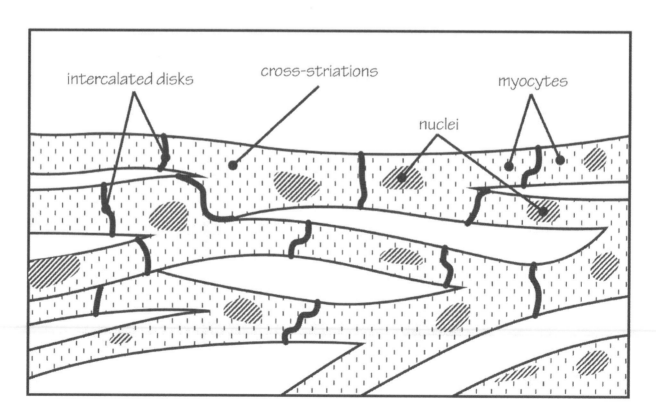

Just outside this muscle layer is the subepicardial layer. It is essentially the connective tissue that attaches the myocardium to the epicardium of the heart.

The epicardium is the outer layer of the heart wall. It is the same thing as the visceral pericardial layer, and is what makes the pericardial lubricating fluid. When you think about the pericardium and its layers, you should recognize that they don't surround the heart. Instead, imagine that the pericardium is a big deflated parachute that drapes over all the surfaces of the heart, so there is the illusion of it surrounding the entire organ, even though embryologically it just began by draping over the heart muscle during development. It explains why there is a thin layer inside and a tougher layer outside.

What does the pericardium do?

The pericardium is an important structure around the heart. It keeps the heart fixed in space, mostly because this covering around the heart is attached to the diaphragm. It's also attached to the great vessels and the sternum overlying the heart. It keeps the heart constrained when it comes to potentially overfilling. The fibrous pericardium is very tough and limits heart movement. Because of the serous layer around the heart, there is effective lubrication as the heart beats, avoiding friction. In some ways, the pericardium also protects the heart from outside infections.

Blood supply to the heart

There are a couple of things to think about when learning about the blood supply to the heart. There are the blood vessels that enter and leave the heart in obvious ways. Certainly you can say that the entirety of your blood supply enters and leaves your heart frequently. In fact, with a normal cardiac output, you shuttle your entire blood supply completely around the loop every single minute. But this isn't the same thing as when we talk about the blood supply to the heart itself, which comes only from the coronary arteries that surround the organ.

As we talk about blood supply, we'll do it in order from just before entering the heart to just after leaving it. As you know now, the process starts when the vessels enter the right atrium, through two large veins known as the inferior and superior vena cava.

The inferior vena cava takes blood from below the diaphragm back to the heart to be pumped into the lungs. Far below this vein are the two common iliac veins in the pelvis, one for draining blood from each leg. There is very little pressure in the venous system, so the veins have valves that help prevent blood from pooling in your feet every time you stand up. Movement of the leg muscles, and thin muscles around the veins, help squeeze blood upward toward the heart.

The superior vena cava takes blood from the upper body, except the heart itself, and sends it to the right atrium. Brachiocephalic veins come together in the thoracic region to drain both sides of the upper body. It comes down along the right side of the chest before entering the heart. You can see in this image that several jugular veins drain the facial and brain areas.

Major veins superior to the heart

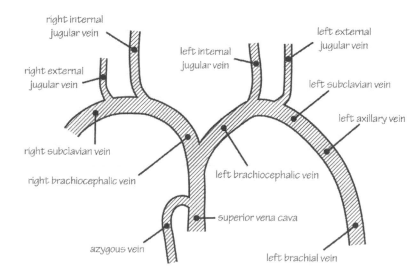

The next main vessel when it comes to blood flowing through the heart is the pulmonary trunk. It comes off the heart as a single vessel, drawing blood out of the right ventricle to each lung. The pulmonary trunk itself is short, quickly separating into the left and right pulmonary arteries. These arteries have many branches getting progressively smaller in diameter until they become capillaries. It's these tiny capillaries that interface in the lungs to collect oxygen and give off carbon dioxide.

This process of gas diffusion in the lungs is largely a matter of physics. The concentration of oxygen gas in the lungs' air sacs or alveoli is higher than the concentration of this gas in the deoxygenated capillaries. This naturally means that oxygen will flow from high-concentration areas to areas of low concentration.

The reverse is true for carbon dioxide. Because of cell metabolism (which gives off CO_2 as a result), the concentration of CO_2 in the veins is higher than in the alveoli. This gas therefore diffuses from the inside of the capillaries into the alveoli proper. This is what gas exchange looks like in these alveoli:

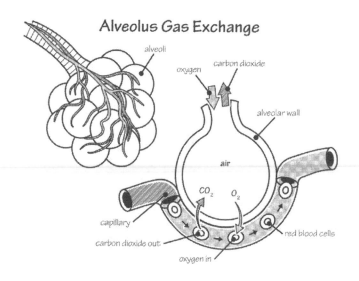

The four major pulmonary veins, two on each side, gather all the blood from the lungs (now oxygenated), drawing it into the left atrium. They do not come together but instead have separate entry points into the left atrium, as shown:

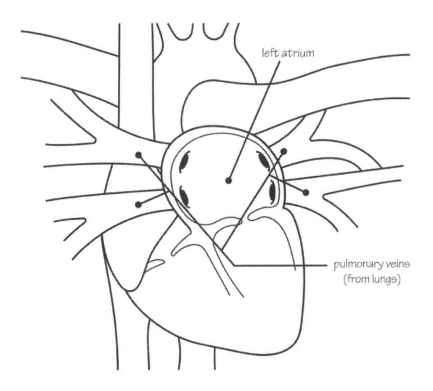

This leaves us with the aorta, which is ready to receive oxygenated blood from the left ventricle so it can go out to the periphery (the systemic circulation) again. Blood is essentially ejected upward for a few inches until it reaches the aortic arch, a true arch that makes a 180-degree turn in order to send blood down to the lower extremities. This arch has its own branches that send blood to the head and neck as well as both upper arms. These major branches look like this:

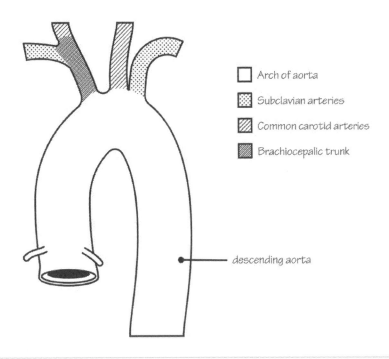

The Coronary Circulation

The coronary circulation is so named because it forms a crown of sorts that surrounds the entire heart. We've talked about how this circulation starts at the sinuses just outside the aortic valve, one opening leading to the heart's right side and the other the left. Here is an anterior (front-on) view of the heart and these major coronary arteries.

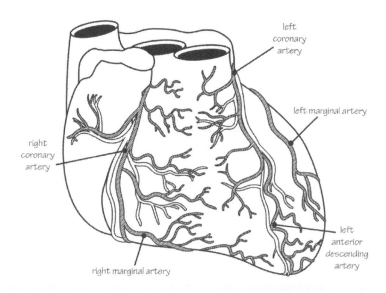

You might think it isn't important to know each of these arteries and which part of the heart they supply, but in fact it is significant and relevant. When you read an ECG and look at the different leads, you will sometimes see specific patterns indicating that one or another artery has been affected or blocked. You must know which arteries are where to determine what a particular pattern of ischemia (or oxygen deficit) means.

As you can see, there is a left and right coronary artery. The left gives rise to three major branches: the anterior descending artery, the circumflex artery, and the marginal artery. About 1 out of 4 of us have an extra branch off the left circumflex artery, called the posterior interventricular artery.

The right coronary artery gives rise to a marginal artery across the right anterior part of the heart, or the posterior interventricular artery in the 1 out of 4 of us who have this artery coming off the left circumflex artery.

So, if you see certain areas of ischemia or heart damage, you should think of these branches possibly being blocked:

- **Anterior surface**—think left anterior descending artery

- **Left anterior surface**—think left marginal artery

- **Left posterior surface**—think circumflex artery

- **Right anterior surface**—think right marginal artery

- **Right posterior surface**—think posterior interventricular artery

- **Inferior surface**—think right marginal artery

This is a rough idea of what this looks like visually:

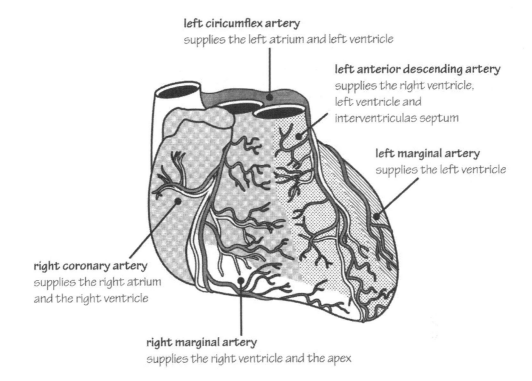

left ciricumflex artery
supplies the left atrium and left ventricle

left anterior descending artery
supplies the right ventricle,
left ventricle and
interventriculas septum

left marginal artery
supplies the left ventricle

right coronary artery
supplies the right atrium
and the right ventricle

right marginal artery
supplies the right ventricle and the apex

Once the blood has supplied the heart structures, it enters the cardiac venous system. Tiny thebesian veins run through the myocardium, taking blood to larger veins outside the heart muscle. These lead into even larger veins that travel along the sulci (alongside the arteries) until they reach the coronary sinus, a large area where blood pools and travels along the coronary sulcus. The coronary sinus empties into the right atrium through a small opening.

Here are the major veins of the heart, including the coronary sinus.

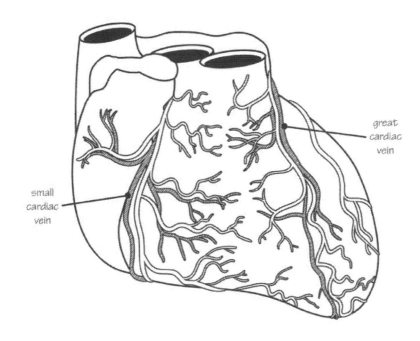

great
cardiac
vein

small
cardiac
vein

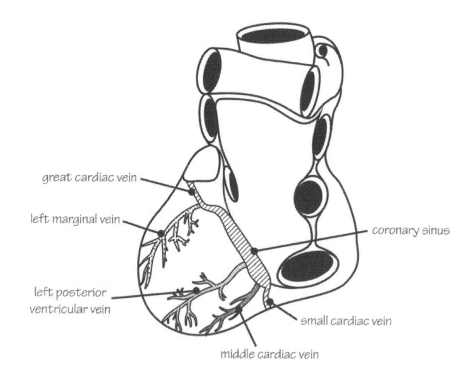

great cardiac vein

left marginal vein

coronary sinus

left posterior
ventricular vein

small cardiac vein

middle cardiac vein

It is not as important to learn the different names of the coronary veins, as these rarely get diseased and aren't a cause of any major ECG changes.

Blood Flow through the Heart Wall

The blood flow through the heart wall itself has one important feature. The major coronary vessels travel along the outside of the heart, but what about the circulation inside the heart itself? It turns out there are perforating arterioles (or extra-small arteries) that punch through the heart wall from outside to inside so that even the endocardium gets blood.

It also means that if there is a slowing or blockage of blood flow in the major coronary arteries, the inner heart wall layers (especially the endocardium and subendocardial areas) are more likely to be shorter on oxygen than the outside of the heart wall.

As you study ECG analysis further, you'll learn how the ECG will show areas of ischemia where there isn't enough oxygen in the heart muscle. You'll hear about "transmural myocardial infarctions" and "subendocardial infarctions." The term "transmural" means all through the heart, while the term "subendocardial" means the damage is confined to the inner heart layers.

You will probably not hear about an "epicardial myocardial infarction" because this isn't likely to happen, since the blood supply is generally much better in this part of the heart. Because the blood flows from outside to inside, you wouldn't have damage to the outer layers of the heart wall without likely having worsened conditions in the inner heart layers at the same time and in the same areas.

The Physiology of the Heart

The heart is not an ordinary pump like you'd find in a non-medical situation. It is a muscle first and foremost, and has a complex circuitry that adjusts in real time to changes in the rest of your body's physiology. A heart that cannot do this is likely to actually be a very sick one. Let's look at the cardiac physiology terms you'll need to understand as you study ECG interpretation.

The Physiology of the Heart Muscle Cell or Myocyte

Heart muscle cells or myocytes have a unique feature not shared by other cells in the body. They have the ability to respond to an electrical signal and generate an "action potential." This causes each muscle to contract as a result. What's unique about them is that they are somewhat "leaky," so they don't keep a normal electrical charge steady at all times. They do not necessarily have to wait until they get a signal from elsewhere in order to contract; and because some electrolytes leak through the cell membrane, they can cause their own action potential without outside influence. This is called *autorhythmicity*.

Before we get into that, let's look at what a resting potential looks like and how it is created. The resting potential of a cell is the electrical charge difference between its inside and outside. Most of this charge difference comes because of the different amounts of charged ions, due to the cells' sodium-potassium ATPase pump that is continually pumping sodium out of the cell and potassium in. Because it sends out three sodium ions for every two potassium ions pumped in, the cell is steadily charged more negatively on the inside, called the *resting potential*. It looks like this:

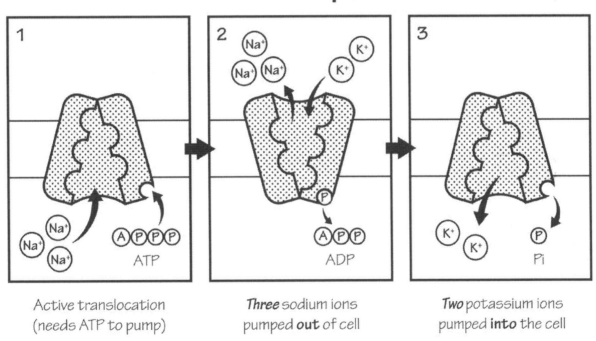

Sodium - Potassium Pump: 3 Na⁺ out ; 2 K⁺ in

Active translocation
(needs ATP to pump)

Three sodium ions
pumped **out** of cell

Two potassium ions
pumped **into** the cell

An action potential for any cell involves a change in the charge differential or voltage across the membrane. Usually it happens when sodium enters the cell, causing more positives inside, called phase 0. Let's look at how this works:

Cardiac Muscle Action Potential

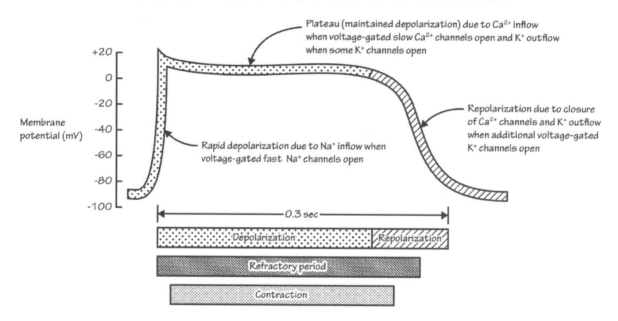

The normal heart muscle cell has a resting potential of about -90 mV across the membrane, being more negative on the inside. This is called phase 4 for some weird reason. Sodium enters the cell in phase 1. This starts the process known as *depolarization*. The sodium ions add a positive charge so that the cell is temporarily positively charged. The charge returning to its resting state is called *repolarization*. This whole process of depolarization and repolarization is called the *action potential*.

There are several different potassium channels in the cell membrane. In phase 4, a series of leaky potassium and calcium channels allow the membrane potential to change slightly. This takes it to a -70 mV state. This inherent leakiness is what triggers the heart muscle cell to spontaneously fire and contract without outside influence.

Then in phase 0, sodium channels open and sodium floods in. The charge in the cell becomes positive at about +50 mV, after which the sodium channels close quickly. Phase 1 then starts, as potassium channels open up to allow potassium to actively leave the cell, driving down the electrical gradient. Phase 2 is when the charge differential plateaus, staying the same because calcium levels become high in the cell to keep the charge positive for a period of time.

After phase 2 ends, the calcium channels close, and calcium is pumped into the cell's sarcoplasmic reticulum. At the same time, potassium leaves the cell in phase 3. This rapidly depolarizes the cell, essentially taking it from its +50 mV state back to its former -90. Of course, it is during this entire time that the cardiac muscle cell contracts.

Cardiomyocyte Contraction

The whole goal of this action potential is to cause muscle contraction. How does this happen? It's similar in some ways to how all muscle cells contract. There are fibers called actin and myosin that slide along each other to shorten the cardiac muscle cell. If you look at it, it appears a lot like this:

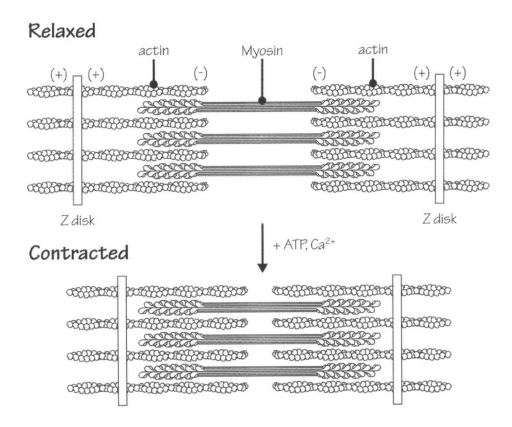

Relaxed

actin   Myosin   actin

(+) (+)   (-)   (-)   (+) (+)

Z disk   Z disk

Contracted   + ATP, Ca²⁺

In the image, you see just one sarcomere, which is a unit of actin and myosin fibers in the cell. There are thousands of sarcomeres lined end to end, and up to 100,000 sarcomeres per muscle fiber in a skeletal muscle fiber, although there is far less cardiac muscle fiber because they are smaller cells.

As you can see, the actin fibers are attached to the Z discs, while the myosin fibers are free (sort of). As the muscle contracts, bridges form between the actin and myosin fibers, where they overlap. The contraction progressively shortens the muscle because the fibers "walk along" each other to shorten the sarcomere.

This whole process takes both calcium ions and ATP energy. Calcium is stored in the sarcoplasmic reticulum of the heart muscle, a fancy name for the cell's endoplasmic reticulum. When the voltage increases inside the cell during depolarization, there are channels in the sarcoplasmic reticulum that respond to the voltage change by releasing the calcium ions, called voltage-gated calcium channels because the "gate" that causes their release is the voltage. This image is what it looks like:

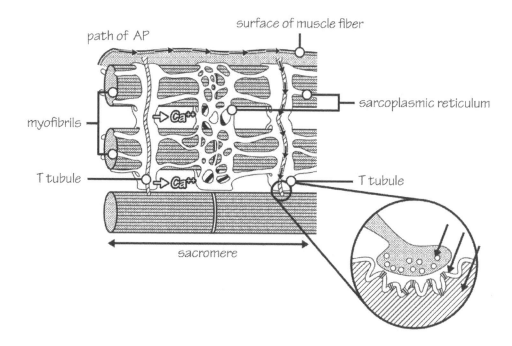

The sarcoplasmic reticulum surrounds each sarcomere so it can quickly release calcium where it is needed. T-tubules extend like pathways for the electrical impulse to come from the cell's outer surface to the deep interior regions where the sarcomeres can be quickly acted on.

Calcium release is essential to muscle contractions of all kinds. You'll see in this image why:

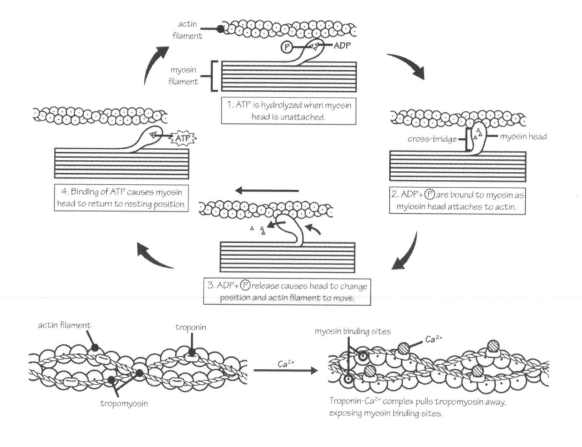

There are two proteins on the actin fiber, called troponin and tropomyosin. These don't bind to myosin, because the tropomyosin is blocking the myosin binding site. Calcium binds to troponin and moves the tropomyosin out of the way. This exposes a binding site on the actin fiber where myosin can attach.

Myosin has an extension coming off of it at certain intervals. This extension binds to the actin, forming a bridge between the two strands. The strands would normally just stay that way except for the fact that ATP energy enters the picture. It causes what's called a "power stroke," where the bridge strokes in one direction to slide the fibers along with each other by just a tiny distance. The cross-bridge then breaks with the help of ATP again. It causes the extension to reattach farther down the line. The whole thing repeats itself regularly until the sarcomere, where the whole muscle fiber shortens noticeably.

To stop the contraction, calcium is pumped back into the sarcoplasmic reticulum. This will cover the actin-binding sites again so that the muscle relaxes.

The Cardiac Pacemaker Cell

There are two different types of muscle cells, which you can think of as "leaders" and "followers." Leader cells are small pacemaker cells that set the rhythm of the heart, called depending on the part the sinoatrial node or SA, atrioventricular node or AV, and a string of cells extending down the interventricular septum and into the ventricles called the bundle of His (atrioventricular bundle) and Purkinje fibers. They are located here:

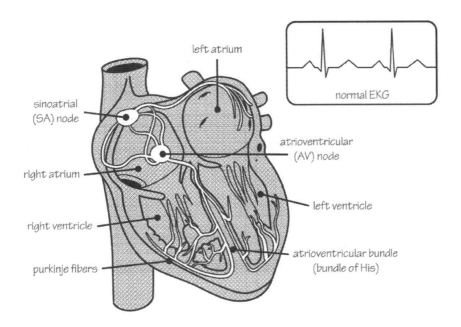

Each of these pacemaker cells has automaticity and the ability to generate their own action potential, but they do it at different rates. The SA node has the fastest rate of automaticity, so it sets the other cells' pace too. If it fails, however, the other cells also have automaticity, but at a slower rate.

The SA node is the main cardiac pacemaker of the heart. Why? Mainly because it has the fastest rate of automaticity. It sets the pace for the rest of the heart, at an average heart rate of 60-100 bpm. When it sends this beat signal to the other parts of the heart's conducting system, it overrides any depolarizations those other parts might themselves have, essentially "conducting the orchestra" and giving no chance for other pacemaker cells to have their own autorhythmicity.

The pathway from the SA node to the AV node is actually several pathways, which is both good and bad. Some heart rhythm problems that typically result in a rapid heart rate come from what's called a reentry rhythm. It involves continual recycling of stimulation to the AV node through a circular pathway in one of these SA-to-AV node pathways.

The heart's electricity's normal pathway is from the SA node to the AV node, to the bundle of His, to the left and right bundle branches, and finally to the Purkinje fibers. If the SA node fails, therefore, the heart does not stop beating altogether. The next area in line (the AV node in this case) will kick in and set its own rhythm. Because they aren't as leaky as the SA node, the AV node cells will cause a slower rate.

The average heart rate generated in each of the main conducting areas of the heart is this:

Normal Activation Sequence	Structure	Conduction velocity (m/sec)	Peacemaker rate (beats/min)
1	SA node	< 0.01	60 -100
2	Atrial myocardium	1.0 - 1.2	None
3	AV node	0.02 - 0.05	40 -55
4	Bundle of His	1.2 - 2.0	25 -40
5	Bundle branches	2.0 - 4.0	25 -40
6	Purkinje network	2.0 - 4.0	25 -40
7	Ventricular myocardium	0.3 - 1.0	None

Cardiac Cycle Events

The cardiac cycle can be thought of in two different ways: as the pathway of blood through the heart, or the pressure changes that happen in the heart. In this section, we will talk about the pressure changes that occur throughout the cardiac cycle.

The two main phases of the cardiac cycle are systole and diastole. In systole, the ventricles contract. Even though the right ventricle has a thinner muscular wall and less strength, it sends the same amount of blood out of it as the left ventricle. It really has to be this way, otherwise blood will pool somewhere in the body, in the lungs or perhaps the systemic circulation. An equal amount for blood needs to flow properly through the entire heart.

Diastole is the time of ventricular filling. The mitral and tricuspid valves both open to allow the atria to contract and push blood into the ventricles. It comes in two phases, and in the second there is an atrial "kick" that pushes as much blood into the ventricles as possible, about 20 percent of the total blood entering the ventricles. This happens immediately before ventricular systole.

In this image, which shows left ventricular pressure, the last rise in diastole comes from the atrial kick (label diastole in the first section and systole in the middle section):

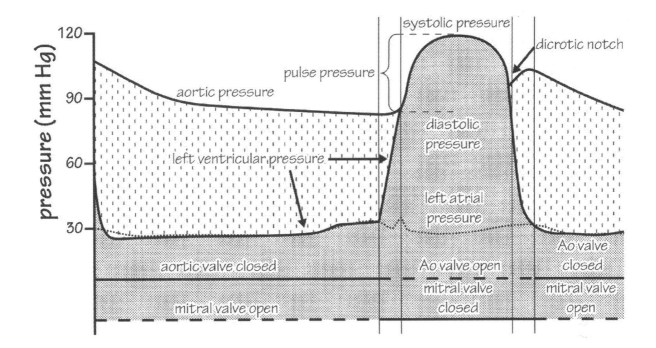

As the ventricle contracts, it isn't the same type the entire time. Pressure changes in the ventricles happen in four phases, called the isovolumic relaxation phase, ventricular filling phase, isovolumic contraction phase, and rapid ventricular ejection phase.

Isovolumic relaxation is when the aortic valve and mitral valve are both closed. The ventricle relaxes but doesn't fill. The mitral valve is induced to open because of this low-pressure situation so blood can flow into the ventricle in the ventricular filling phase. As the ventricle contracts first, both the mitral and aortic valves are closed. As the ventricular ejection phase starts, the aortic valve (and this valve only) opens, so that blood can leave the heart itself.

The maximum and minimum pressures in the heart chambers are these:

- Left ventricle—15 to 120 mm Hg

- Right ventricle—5 to 25 mm Hg

- Right atria—4 to 5 mm Hg

- Pulmonary arteries and left atria—10 to 25 mm Hg

- Aorta 80 to 120 mm Hg

Preload, Afterload, and Contractility

The terms "preload" and "afterload" are confusing terms in heart physiology, but are nevertheless important to understand. They are pressure numbers that happen at certain stages of the cardiac cycle. This is a basic look at preload and afterload:

Preload and Afterload

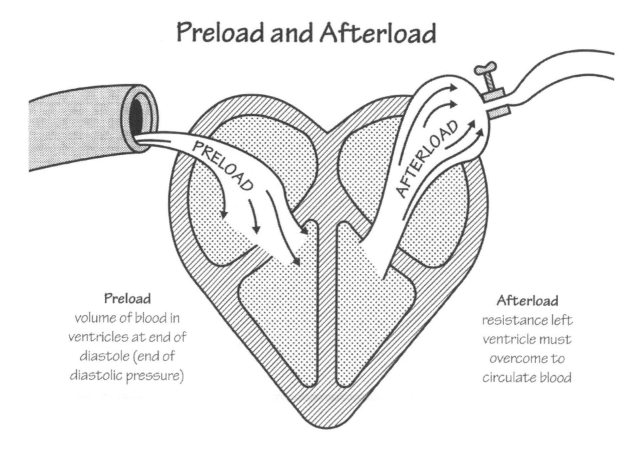

Preload
volume of blood in ventricles at end of diastole (end of diastolic pressure)

Afterload
resistance left ventricle must overcome to circulate blood

Preload is also called the LVEDP, or left ventricular end-diastolic pressure. It is a measure of how much the ventricular wall is stretched at the end of diastole. Preload influences several things, including the stroke volume (how much blood is ejected from each ventricle during systole) and the cardiac output (the amount of blood the heart pumps per minute). It also influences how the heart functions.

As the preload or pressure increases, the heart muscle fibers stretch normally, and there is tension on the muscle wall. However, the muscle will contract normally in the heart, so that the heart's output will be normal in a non-diseased heart.

The Frank-Starling curve was designed by two physiologists, Otto Frank and Ernest Henry Starling, who looked at what happens to the heart if preload is increased. They looked at the extremes of too-low and too-high preloads. Their work led to this curve, which looks at the pressures in the ventricle:

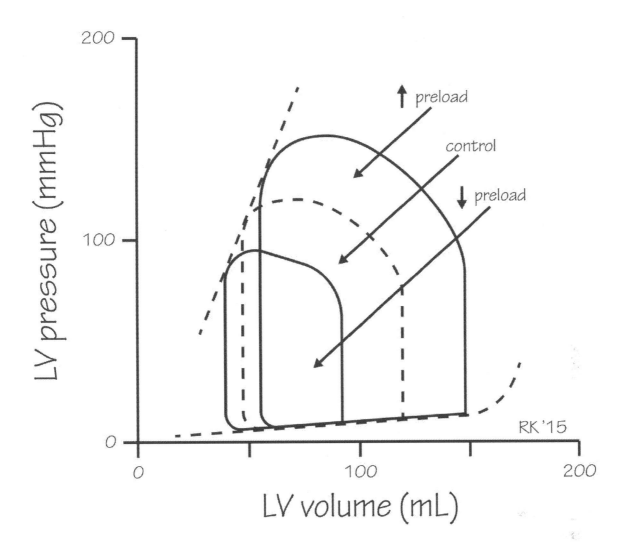

LV pressure (mmHg) vs LV volume (mL) graph with labels: ↑ preload, control, ↓ preload. RK '15

In heart failure, if the left ventricular volume is too high, it will lead to a boggy heart that doesn't contract in a normal way. The stroke volume is the total area under the curve. When the ventricular volume is high, the stroke volume isn't as robust as it should be.

How do you measure the preload? You can introduce a catheter and measure the pulmonary capillary wedge pressure. This measures the pressure in a small pulmonary artery that is occluded by the catheter. This measures the back pressure from the left atrium, because there is no valve or pressure gradient between them. This pressure measurement correlates to preload.

The afterload is best described as the force that opposes the ejection of blood from the heart. This is calculated as the total force opposing the heart muscle's contraction, minus the heart's existing force before the contraction, essentially the load or pressure the heart must push against. You can't really know what this value is for sure, because it depends on the ventricular shape over time, so we use arterial pressure or blood pressure as a substitute measure.

The afterload affects the end-systolic volume in the ventricles, the left end-diastolic pressure, and the stroke volume. This is just like the fuel injector of your car, ejecting fuel to propel itself. If there is a blockage or if the tube leading out of the injector is too narrow, it will be harder for the injector to do its job. In the case of your heart, your cardiac output will fall, mostly because there isn't enough blood pushing out of the heart with each beat.

The Frank-Starling curve looks at the effect of changes in afterload on the heart function. The higher the afterload, the greater the chance that the heart gives out and the person goes into "heart failure," which is a lot like pump failure of any pump that is overworked:

Healthy Heart Compared to Cardiac Failure

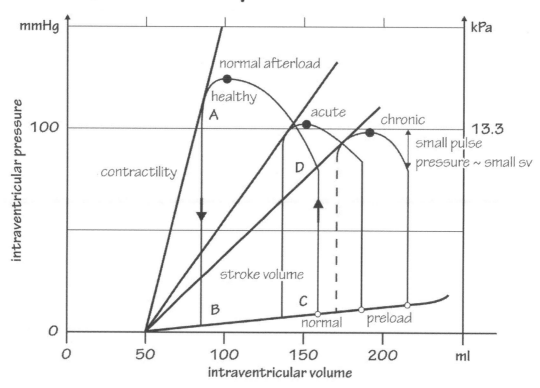

Notice the lines on the last curve that measures "contractility." This is also called inotropy, which is the strength of each contraction. A poorly contracting heart does not shorten its fibers when the contraction is happening; essentially, the heart is weaker than it should be. This is common in many types of heart failure.

How we measure heart performance:

One of the measures of heart function is called the cardiac output, or how much blood the heart puts out per minute. This is an easy calculation if you have an echocardiogram (an ultrasound of the heart) that measures how much blood is ejected from the heart per beat. It's only the amount ejected from the left ventricle that counts, known as stroke volume. Multiply this by the heart rate per minute and you get the cardiac output. It looks like this:

Cardiac Output (CO) = Heart rate (HR) X Stroke volume (SV)

CO = HR x End diastolic volume - End systolic volume

CO is about 4 to 5 liters per minute at rest

EF (ejection fraction) = % of End diastolic volume ejected with each beat

EF = 50 to 70 percent in normal people

If the heart has poor contractility, it will be like a boggy sac and have a poor ability to push blood out. You will often note a high end-diastolic volume and a low ejection fraction, which is the percent of blood pumped out of a filled ventricle with each heartbeat. This is because such a large and boggy heart simply can't contract well enough to push blood out of the ventricles. But the good news is that the cardiac output increases dramatically with exercise.

Transmission of Electrical Impulses

Electrical activity is a natural property of biological cells, although "electricity" is not really the right term here. In reality it is electrochemistry we talk about when dealing with the electricity of the body. This means that the electricity comes from ions that are themselves electrically charged. When ions move from one place to another, usually across a membrane or down a membrane, this is where the electricity comes from.

Even though it is chemical electricity, it can still be measured. It is why the ECG can pick up the electrical signals from the heart, because you can pick up such signals from nerve cells and muscle cells too. An electromyogram picks up the electricity that comes from the muscle cells, and a nerve conduction study picks up the electrical flow through a nerve. An EEG or electroencephalogram measures the electrical patterns in the brain.

There are charged molecules throughout the body, but the ones that participate in nerve and muscle cells' electrical activity are mainly ions, usually charged atoms or small molecules. The ones you might be most familiar with are electrolytes. When you measure a person's electrolytes, you usually measure the sodium, potassium, chloride, and bicarbonate levels. Calcium is an ion that is also essential in the heart, mostly because it is necessary for the heart muscle to contract.

Let's look again at the action potential to see what we mean by absolute and refractory heart muscle contraction periods. An absolute refractory period is when the heart muscle cell can't be reactivated to make another action potential. This is a good thing, because it means the heart can't just go wild and beat whenever it wants. You need this refractory period to prevent serious heart rhythm disturbances or "arrhythmias." This image shows when the absolute refractory period is during the action potential:

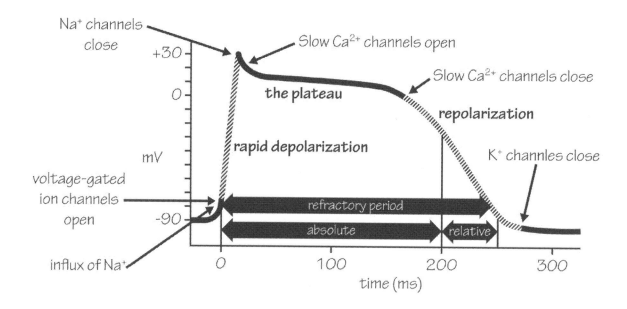

The absolute refractory period is a pause button on the heart muscle's ability to be restimulated to contract again, expressed as the amount of time it takes. During the absolute refractory period, the cell membrane's sodium and calcium channels are inactive, so it is impossible to start another action potential.

The difference between the absolute and relative refractory periods is easy to remember. The absolute refractory period is when it is impossible to have any new action potential, while the relative refractory period is when there is a possibility that a new action potential could happen, but it would be harder to do. This period occurs right after an action potential moves down the axon, so it would have to occur by a larger than normal stimulus.

The image doesn't show that when potassium exits the cell to cause repolarization, there is a period called **hyperpolarization**. It's when the potassium overshoots the goal and causes too much electronegativity in the cell. The cell could still depolarize during this time, but it would take a larger stimulus in order to do this. When the resting potential returns to normal, the relative refractory period ends.

It isn't shown in the above image because it represents a regular muscle cell's action potential; but in pacemaker cells in the heart, such as the SA node, the action potential looks different. It has a certain threshold of -40 mV that triggers the action potential to happen. Before this, there are the leaky sodium channels, also called "funny sodium channels," that slowly leak sodium into the cell. When it reaches the magic threshold, both sodium and calcium rapidly enter the cell through different channels.

The repolarization happens with a fast outflow of potassium out of the cell. These cells don't need a long break, as you see with the heart's cardiomyocytes' drawn-out action potential, because they don't contract, although they do hyperpolarize as you can see (where the line drops below the threshold). These funny sodium channels start up and pace the cell's electrical output by leaking sodium back into the pacemaker cell.

SA Node Potentials

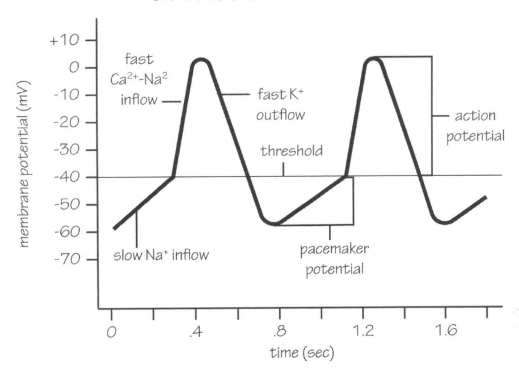

Funny channels are called that because they leak both sodium and potassium at different times. These channels flow in what's called the "pacemaker" current, because they set the cell's pacemaker activity and are the whole reason the heart has inherent automaticity (that is, the ability to regulate itself without outside influence).

What the ECG Signals Mean

Before we talk about what the ECG signals mean on a small scale, you should review what happens as the heart's electrical system functions in real time. As you know, in a healthy person, the SA node starts initiating a heartbeat because it has the fastest rate of automaticity. It sends that signal across the atria, signaling these muscles to contract. As you can imagine, this starts blood flowing through the ventricles as they fill during diastole.

The electrical signal also reaches the AV node. This node is critical because there is a pause or delay in the passage onward of the electrical signal here. If you know how the heart works, you'll see why this is important. If the signal reached the ventricles too fast, they would contract before they had a chance to fill up with blood. The whole thing would be out of sync. The resting period or delay in the AV node helps allow for this filling up of the ventricles, lasting about 120 milliseconds (ms).

After the AV node, the signal goes down the bundle of His and splits into the left and right bundle branches. Then they travel in a wide array around the ventricles through the Purkinje fibers. As you can see, these will cause the ventricles to squeeze upward like a tube of toothpaste, to send blood up to the semilunar valves and outside the heart itself.

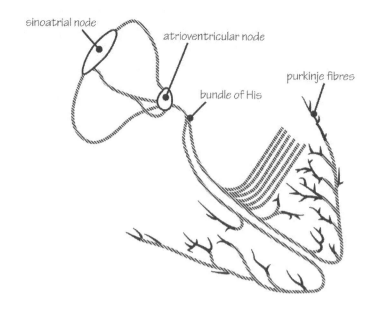

See how coordinated the whole thing is? It is truly a symphony of electrical activity and contractions that allow blood to effectively flow through the heart and eject from it.

Did you know? *Artificial pacemakers are used to keep the heart going at a regular pace when it can't do it by itself. A wire is passed into the heart through the veins leading to the organ, then inserted into the heart muscle. It paces the heart by sending regular signals for it to contract. It works best for slow heartbeats or "bradycardia," and is harder to be effective for fast heartbeats or "tachycardia," because the pacemaker has difficulty interrupting a faster rate than its own. Remember that the fastest pacemaker to the heart "wins," and therefore sets the overall heart rate.*

Now we get to the interesting stuff about what happens to the heart's electrical activity during a single beat. It is the electrical activity you'll see every time you read an ECG, and we will talk a lot more about this in a minute. But first, here is what the typical electrical activity looks like in a single heartbeat:

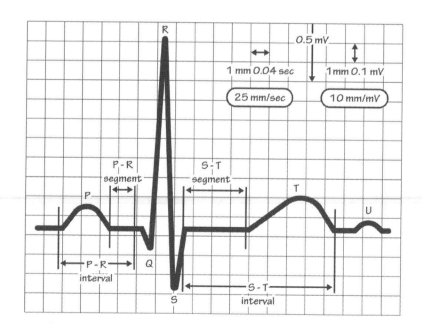

The paper used on an ECG is designed so that each tiny 1 mm square in width equals 0.04 seconds, and each 1 mm in height stands for 0.1 millivolts in electrical activity. This means that the strip outputs at a pace of 25 millimeters per second, and that 10 millimeters (1 cm) equals one millivolt.

The beat starts with a P wave, representing the electrical activity you'll see when the atria depolarize or begin to contract. The space between the beginning of the P wave and the start of the next wave (the R wave) is called the PR interval. This represents atrial depolarization to the beginning of ventricular depolarization or contraction. Within there is an even smaller part called the PR segment, which is the space between the end of the P wave and the start of the R wave.

The QRS complex is next. It starts with a slight downward deflection called the Q wave, then peaks upward to make a deflection called the R wave. Then it drops sharply down to the S wave before moving back up to the baseline. The width of the QRS complex is important in knowing if the AV node is working right. It should be relatively narrow. It reflects the time of ventricular depolarization.

Hidden inside the QRS complex is the repolarization wave. This means the atria are returning to a resting state wave of the atria. You can't actually see it because the QRS complex hides it.

After the QRS complex is the ST segment between the S peak and the beginning of the T wave. The ST interval isn't as important clinically, but is the interval between the S peak and the end of the T wave. The T wave represents the time of ventricular repolarization or the ventricles returning to a state of rest.

Not everyone has a U wave; it is usually an abnormal finding in the heart. It is a tiny wave that is thought to occur when the Purkinje fibers depolarize, but really no one knows this for sure.

This next image shows what is happening in the cardiac cycle during a single cycle. The artificial beginning of the cycle is during both atrial diastole and ventricular diastole. The P wave is the electrical beginning of the cardiac cycle. Note that the start of both the atria and ventricles' systole happens essentially at the peak of the P wave and QRS complex respectively. This is because these parts of the heart muscle need the electrical impulse first before they can contract.

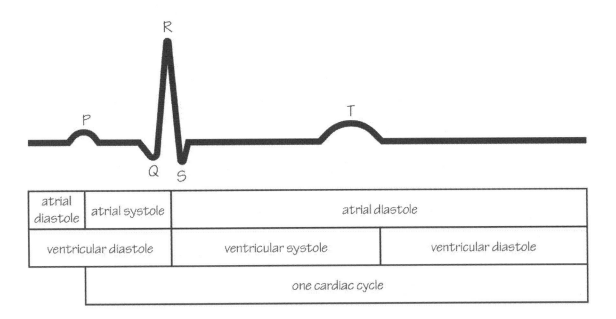

Innervation of the Heart

To be sure, the heartbeat is capable of beating by itself with nothing more than a good blood supply. If this weren't possible, you could never have a heart transplant, since with transplants of any kind including the heart, you don't ever connect the nerves. Instead, without nerves the "denervated" transplanted heart still beats at about 90 to 100 bpm by itself.

Let's see how the normal heart operates. In the medulla oblongata or lower brainstem, there are nuclei (collections of nerve cell bodies) that regulate the heart rate. These contain the nerve cells for the autonomic nervous system. This system has two major branches, the sympathetic and parasympathetic.

The sympathetic nervous system is the "fight or flight" system of the heart, which causes it to beat more rapidly—just as you would notice if you were suddenly frightened by something. The parasympathetic nervous system has the opposite effect, slowing the heart rate.

There are nerves for both of these branches that attach to the heart to influence the heart rate. You may have heard of the vagus nerve. It is the tenth cranial nerve and the main supplier of parasympathetic nervous system activity to the heart. When it influences the heart to slow it down, this is called the "vagal brake" acting on the heart.

The process isn't entirely automatic, because you can purposely think of a scary thing and cause your heart to race. Your thoughts come from the cortex and travel through the hypothalamus and to the medulla oblongata. This will activate the sympathetic or parasympathetic branches in order to affect your heart rate and blood pressure. But it can happen without thinking as well, because you can sense danger from your body without full conscious thought. Such a thing also will influence the brainstem and affect your heart rate and blood pressure.

The brainstem's two main nuclei are the nucleus tractus solitarius (NTS) or solitary nucleus, which gets influenced by chemical receptors, as well as ones called baroreceptors that monitor your blood pressure. When this gets activated, it turns off the rostral ventrolateral medulla's nucleus to put out sympathetic nervous activity.

The parasympathetic neurons in the dorsal vagal nucleus and the nucleus ambiguous (also in the medulla) get activated by the NTS. They trigger the activity of the tenth cranial nerve, slowing the heart rate significantly. The heart always has some vagal brake from this nerve all the time, so that the actual normal heart rate is less than the "denervated setpoint" of about 100 beats per minute.

The hypothalamus also has a role in all this. If you are stressed from exercise or excessive heat, for example, this will stress the sympathetic nervous system in order to speed the heart rate. It will also occur if you are sick or anxious.

There are a couple of terms you should know concerning the heart and its innervation, including:

- **Chronotropy**. This is related to the heart rate itself, and essentially means anything that can change it. A positive chronotropic agent will speed up the heart, while a negative chronotropic agent will slow it down.

- **Inotropy**. This refers to the strength or force of the contraction. Some drugs will increase the heart's inotropy, and others will decrease it.

- **Dromotropy**. This refers to the velocity of electricity through the cardiac conduction system. Sympathetic influence on the heart will increase the heart's dromotropy, while parasympathetic influence will decrease it. Various medications can positively and negatively affect the heart's dromotrophy.

There is regular innervation of the heart that has nothing to do with the autonomic nervous system. This comes from the phrenic nerve, which emerges from the neck at the cervical root 3, 4, and third through fifth cervical vertebral areas. This provides sensory and motor innervation to the pericardium and diaphragm. It can often cause chest pain that isn't coming from the heart itself, but instead is a referred pain that only feels like it.

To Sum Things Up

You now know a lot more about the heart than perhaps you've ever learned before. It is a vital organ necessary for our survival. Its main job is to pump blood to the lungs for oxygenation, and then pump the oxygenated blood to the rest of the body. It has two atrial chambers that receive blood and two ventricular chambers that eject blood.

The heart's electrical system or "conduction system" is how the heart can regulate the contractions in a specific way. There is the main pacemaker of the heart called the sinoatrial node or SA node. The signal it creates gets sent to all parts of the heart in a specific pattern. As each heart muscle fiber or cardiomyocyte gets activated, the heart will contract in a unified fashion to allow it to act as a functional syncytium, which squeezes blood out like you'd squeeze a tube of toothpaste.

CHAPTER 2:
VECTORS, ACTUAL ECG, AND ECG TOOLS

Before we get too deep in what each ECG defection wave means, we should first look more deeply into how ECGs work and what the different types look like. What are electrodes and leads? What is the ECG axis all about? How do you perform an ECG anyway, and figure it out too? We will look at these things comprehensively, so you will be able to look at any ECG and read much more into it than the series of squiggles they might look like to you now.

Working with vectors

Before we get too far into ECG analysis, we should first understand the relationship ECGs have with vectors. What is a vector? It's a certain value or number that has a direction to it. In chemistry and biology, we sometimes call these "dipoles," because they are related to electrical vectors and not mathematical vectors.

A written vector is a picture resembling an arrow of what the number value looks like. Like any arrow, it will be a certain length; the longer it is, the bigger the number value. It will have a certain direction too, which indicates the direction the number value is pointing. A simple vector looks like this:

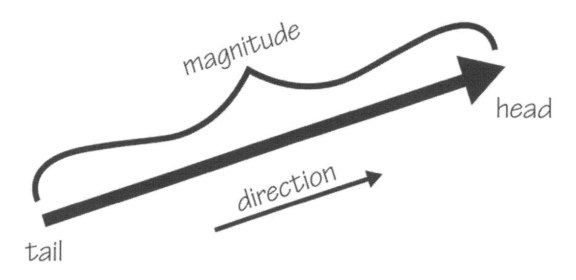

An arrow like this makes no sense if you don't put it in context. If you put a vector on a graph, however, suddenly you have the context you're looking for:

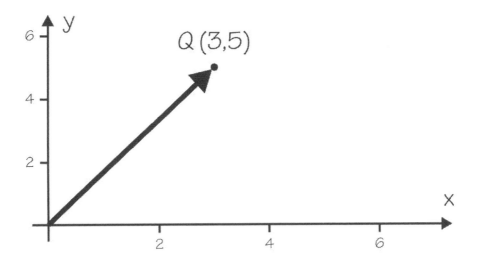

It can help to put a vector on a graph so you can see it in context. Another way to do it is to imagine a 360-degree circle. You know that zero degrees are straight to the right, and 180 degrees is straight to the left. Now you can describe a vector as having a length, with a number value representing an angle on a 360-degree circle. See all those vectors?

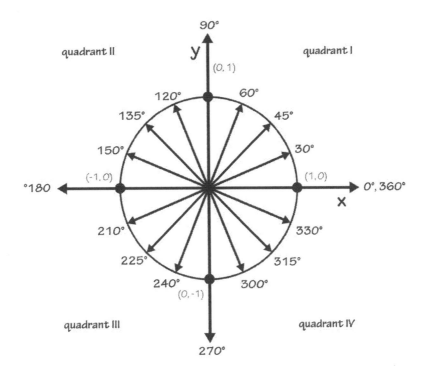

You aren't a 2D person in real life but are instead three-dimensional, so you have to add a third axis (the z-axis) to represent that. The good news is that you can say a lot about an ECG even if you don't picture the heart or even your body as 3D.

Vectors are added differently than regular numbers. Usually if you have three numbers, like 2 + 4 + 3, you can just add them to get 9. If these are vectors, though, they don't add up in the same way, because the direction matters.

For example, let's picture two vectors on a graph called "a" and "b." In reality, these are just names of vectors and not the vectors themselves; the real vectors are called (a1, a2) and (b1, b2). The a1 and b1 are the part of the vector in the x-direction, while the a2 and b2 represent the y-direction. Adding them is a matter of adding the 1s and the 2s separately to get the final vector. It looks graphically like this:

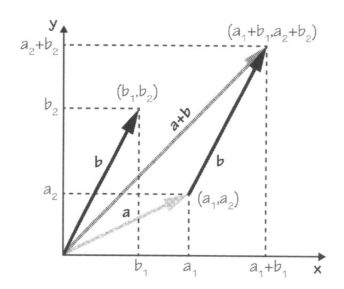

You can do it graphically by putting the vectors head to tail as long as you keep each vector's actual direction intact as you do this. The graph shown above helps you see how you can get the final vector as it looks pictorially.

On the ECG, the image you see on the paper is two-dimensional, but it doesn't represent two dimensions at all. You perceive these wave patterns as they look in two dimensions, but in reality they are three-dimensional.

The ECG involves electrical vectors because they too have a number value (the electrical charge), plus a direction for that charge to go. You measure charge in volts, millivolts, or something similar. In the ECG, zero millivolts are called the "isoelectric line," and you'll see deflections above and below that line.

When you ponder the 3D vectors in the ECG, you can think of three directions: positive, negative, or zero. Electricity traveling to the positive electrode means the vector and voltage will be positive, while going to the negative electrode means negative. If you measured the vector perpendicular (at a 90-degree angle) to the direction of the charge, you would get a zero recording, because no part of the charge is going in that direction at all.

If you are thoroughly confused by now, don't be disheartened. You will see soon how all of this applies to reading an ECG, and begin making sense of what you are seeing.

How does the ECG work?

The heart, as you know now, depolarizes and repolarizes on a cell-by-cell basis. Each individual cell doesn't contribute much to the total picture, but when you add up these electrical changes to include the entire heart muscle, you can get a much bigger electrical change you can physically see.

So how can you get an idea of the electrical activity of the heart through the skin, like how ECGs work? Well, you are an electrical conductor yourself, mainly because so much of you is water and salt. Saltwater conducts electricity nicely, so you can "see" the heart's electrical activity virtually transmitted throughout your body.

By necessity, the ECG must be very sensitive. You're not a lightbulb, after all; there's only one millivolt or so going through your body, not the 120 volts a lightbulb gives off! The electricity is picked up through electrodes or patches on the skin, which can detect subtle electrical changes that have made their way to these far-flung parts of your body through its saltwater.

As you'll see, the electrodes are attached to "leads," which are ways to see the activity based on calculations of electricity differences picked up on the different electrodes. For example, bipolar leads compare the electrical patterns seen on one limb compared to another.

Of course, most people have four limbs, but to read an ECG you have to consider only three of them: two arms but just one leg. The major bipolar leads in the heart are numbered I, II and III. They look graphically like this:

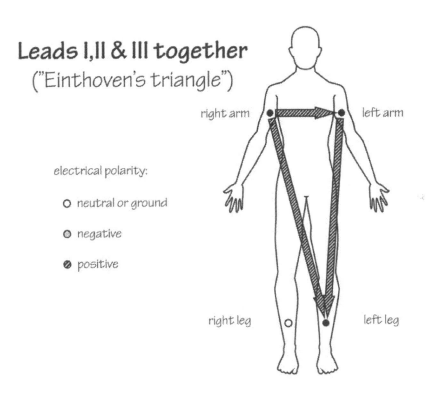

The triangle you see is totally imaginary. The right leg is called "the ground" or electrically neutral. With electricity, you have to have some kind of baseline in which to compare other electrical patterns. The right-arm-to-left-arm lead is numbered I and goes to the right. The right-arm-to-left-leg lead is II and goes down and to the left. Lead III is a left-arm-to-left-leg vector that goes down and to the right.

Did you know? *Willem Einthoven was a Dutch physiologist who studied ECGs at the turn of the twentieth century. He used saltwater pails and put the "victim's" hands and foot into them in place of using actual electrodes. In the end, the results were good enough that he won the 1924 Nobel Prize for Physiology and Medicine for his work on early ECG machines.*

Your ECG interpretation will also depend on what are called V leads. These help to put the whole ECG-reading process into a three-dimensional sphere. There are six of these scattered across the chest's front; they are called V1 through V6. We will chat later about how to place the electrodes to monitor these leads, but essentially they look like this:

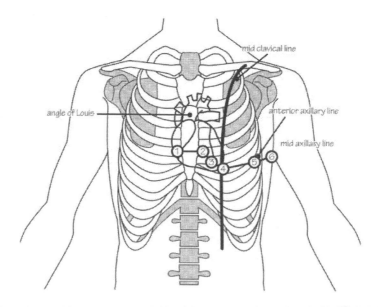

We no longer confine ourselves to the simple leads that Einthoven used. There are several others used in the standard 12-lead ECG.

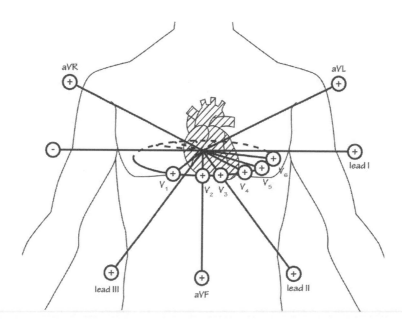

These days you have the same three leads Einthoven used (I, II, and III), but now you also have three more (aVR, aVL, and aVF), called augmented leads. aVR points to the right at 30 degrees above the horizontal, aVL points to the left at 30 degrees above the horizontal, and aVF points straight down toward the foot.

The V leads are vectors spread out over a horizontal circle around the heart. They are smaller vectors in appearance and give you a better idea of the heart's three-dimensional properties. As you can see, the first few (V1 through V3) are better able to tell you what's happening in the anterior or front of the heart, while the last few (V4 through V6) can show you what's happening on the left lateral side of the heart. If you've been doing your math, you can now see where they got the concept of the 12-lead ECG. There are six limb leads, and six "precordial" or V leads.

The virtual leads (aVR, aVL, and aVF) are based on a common virtual electrode known as Wilson's central terminal, or the Vw electrode. It represents the averages of the existing electrodes you already know (RA, LL, and LA), sitting arbitrarily in the center of the body. All in one place, they officially look like this:

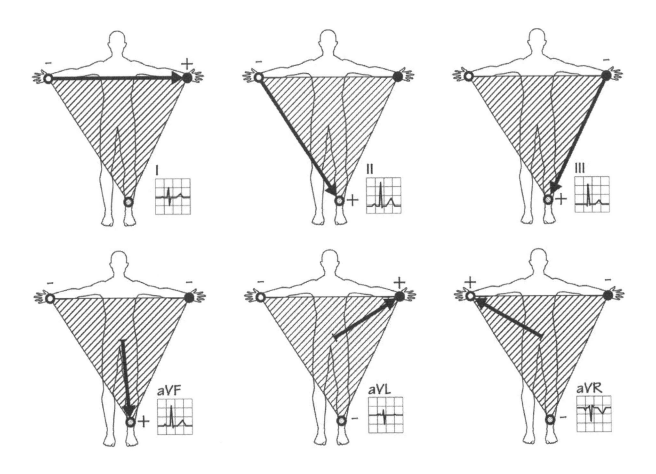

There are also specialized leads used for diagnostic reasons. These include right-sided leads used to look specifically at anything that might be wrong with the right ventricle, also used to evaluate a person with dextrocardia (where the heart is a mirror image in its shape and position compared to normal people). Right atrial arrhythmias are studied with a Lewis lead; in this case, you would place the electrode along the right sternal border at the level of the second intercostal space.

Other specialized leads involve those where an esophageal electrode is placed inside the esophagus itself. The idea is to get a clearer picture of rhythm disturbances like atrial flutter, or atrioventricular reentry disturbances. Rarely, doctors can get an intracardiac ECG using internal electrodes that gather information about the heart right from the source, using a catheter inserted into the heart's chambers.

Electrodes and Waves

We've talked about the leads so far, but not about the electrodes you use to get the actual ECG tracing. Electrodes are small conductive pads often moistened with a water-based gel, used to pick up the heart's electrical activity as it looks by the time it gets to the different parts of the skin. They measure the difference in electrical potential between two arbitrary points on the body.

There are two main classes of electrodes. The circular ones have adhesive on the edges and a gel pad in the middle. These stick longer than other types of electrodes, so they are good for times when you want to keep them on for a long time, like with ambulatory ECG readings. The flat ones are square or rectangular. They stick on nicely for a brief period of time and are used for basic short-term ECG readings.

The gel on each of these electrodes conducts electricity, and usually has silver and silver chloride in it to help it conduct electrons, as they pass from the patient's skin to the wire that leads to the ECG machine.

You will compare the electrode on the right arm to one on the left to get the value of lead I, which is the vector we've been talking about with a magnitude related to the charge differential you get between the two electrodes. All of the leads, then, are nothing but comparisons between the points of the electrodes placed.

However, you have six leads throughout the chest (pericardial electrodes), but only have electrodes on the four extremities. So how do you get all of these extra leads? It's because some aren't literal but virtual, calculated based on averaging the electricity of the physical electrodes you already do have placed.

Did you know? While some ECG techs say, "I'm going to put these leads on you," they don't really mean that, as you have hopefully figured out. The electrode is the spot you put on the skin. The leads are the vectors you create by placing the electrodes on the skin. It is important to remember that the terms "electrode" and "lead" do not mean the same thing.

This image shows you where you place your limb electrodes more specifically. Note that you don't have to put the limb electrodes on the most distal part of the arms or legs, but can put them near the shoulders and upper legs, and get the same result, as long as you stay consistent and put all leads on in the same way (proximal or distal but not both):

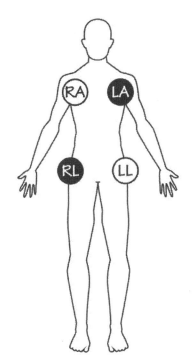

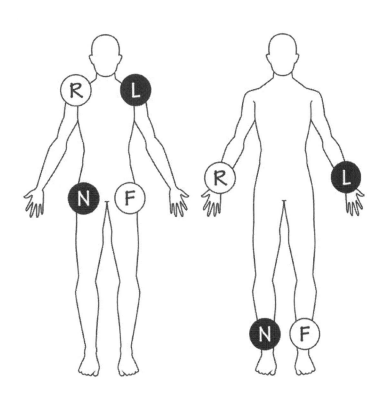

The chest electrodes, labeled V1 through V2, are placed in these areas:

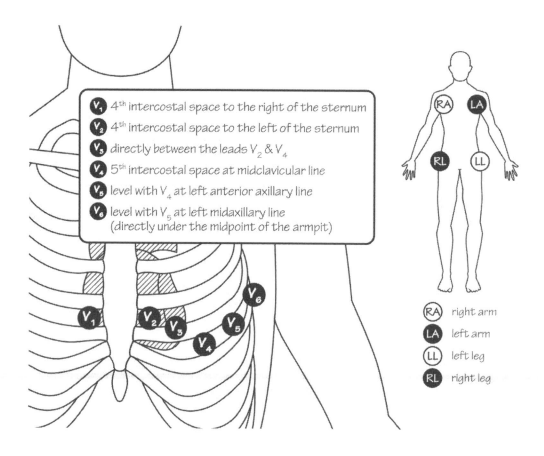

This amounts to a total of ten electrodes, color-coded in standard ways by the American Heart Association so you can visualize where you should put them:

Limb Electrodes

- Left am (LA): black
- Right arm (RA): white
- Left foot or leg (F): red
- Right foot or leg (N for "neutral"): green

Chest or Precordial Electrodes

- V1—in the fourth intercostal space on the right side of the sternum (red)
- V2—in the fourth intercostal space on the left side of the sternum (yellow)
- V3—in the space midway through V2 and V4 (green)
- V4—in the fifth intercostal space along the midclavicular line (blue or brown)
- V5—along the anterior axillary line at the same level as V4 (orange or black)
- V6—along the midaxillary line at the same level as V5 or in the axilla (purple)

For people with pronounced breasts (such as most women, for example), you should place the chest electrodes beneath the breasts and not on top of them.

Electrical axis of the heart

This leads us to the topic of an axis. You probably know, for example, that the Earth is tilted on its axis. How do you define this axis if the Earth is just a sphere floating in space? You can only do it if you have some point of reference. The early astronomers set the reference point as the plane of the planet's orbit around the sun. The Earth is tilted because its north and south poles sit crookedly compared to this plane of reference. It looks like this:

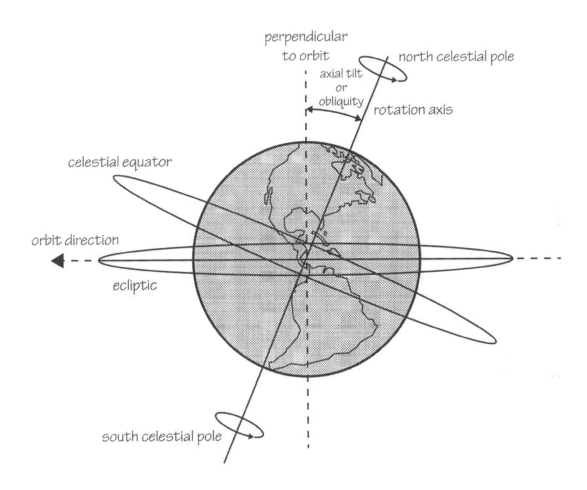

The heart isn't exactly a sphere in space, but it is three dimensional and still needs a reference point. It has therefore been set off to the patient's right and in a horizontal direction. But because we're talking about electricity, you need to think of the axis a bit differently. The heart axis is what you'd get if you averaged all the directions of the different vectors. Translated into electrical terms, it means the direction in which most of the electricity is traveling inside the heart.

To be clear, the axis is two-dimensional. It's based on the limb leads but not the V leads or precordial leads. When you look at the axis of the heart, it's a lot like the 360-degree circle, but now you can see where the leads are located. Note the picture places zero degrees on the right-hand side of the page, but it's actually on the person's left-hand side. The arrows you see are always positive in the direction the arrowhead is pointing. Do you notice how it divides the circle into 30-degree segments?

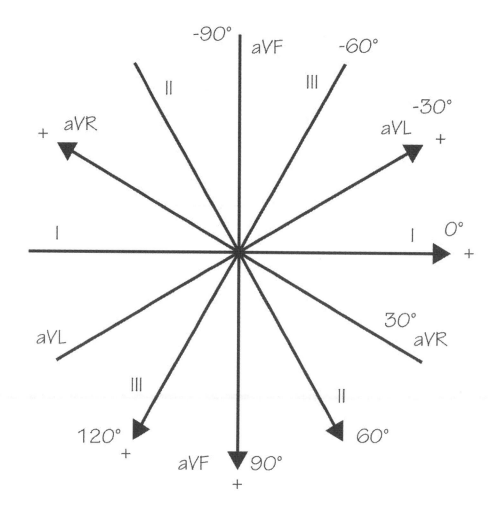

As you move clockwise from lead I, you get a positive axis. If you go counterclockwise, you get a negative axis. It's a total wash once you get back to the start of lead I.

What does it mean when we say the "axis is deviated?" A normal heart axis is anywhere between -30 degrees and +90 degrees. If you get too far north of that on the patient's left, you get left axis deviation, or rarely extreme left axis deviation. If you instead go to the patient's right past +90 degrees to 180 degrees, this is called right axis deviation. It looks a lot like this:

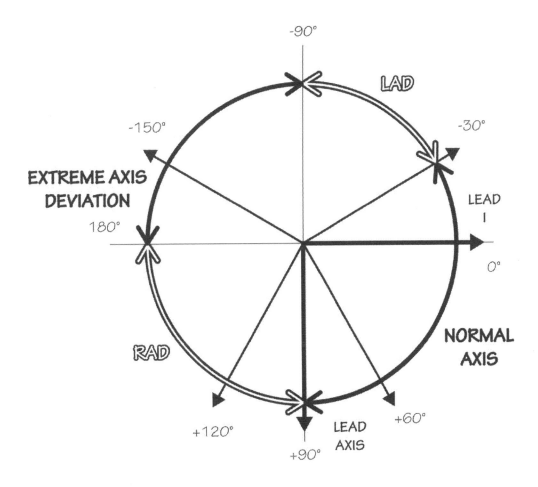

Now we will look at how you determine if a patient's axis is deviated in one direction or another. There are simple ways to get an idea of the axis, and more specific and particular ways. The easiest way is to look only at the deflection of the QRS complex you see in leads I, II and III on a standard 12-lead ECG. It looks like this:

Lead	Normal Axis	Right Axis Deviation	Left Axis Deviation
Lead I	Positive deflection of QRS complex	Negative deflection of QRS complex	Positive deflection of QRS complex
Lead II	Positive deflection of QRS complex	Positive or negative deflection	Negative deflection of QRS complex
Lead III	Positive or negative deflection	Positive deflection of QRS complex	Negative deflection of QRS complex

Another quick way is to look only at leads I and aVF to see if they are mostly positive or negative. Remember that lead I is straight to the patient's left, and lead aVF is straight to the patient's feet. What you get looks like this:

Lead I Deflection	Lead aVF Deflection	Axis Quadrant	Axis Degree
POSITIVE	POSITIVE		Normal Axis of 0 degrees to 90 degrees
POSITIVE	NEGATIVE		Left Axis Deviation of 0 degrees to -90 degrees
NEGATIVE	POSITIVE		Right Axis Deviation of +90 degrees to +180 degrees
NEGATIVE	NEGATIVE		Extreme Axis Deviation of -90 degrees to -180 degrees

We will talk later about how to do this more specifically, even though you usually don't need a specific axis number. Knowing the axis is important in understanding and identifying various cardiac disorders, including congenital heart diseases, ventricular enlargement, conduction defects, and certain types of tachycardias.

Types of ECGs

There are three main types of ECGs, which differ in what they are used for:

- **Resting ECG**. This is the typical ECG you perform on a supine and resting patient. The usual complete version of the resting ECG is 12-lead, but there are single lead, 3-lead, and 5-lead subtypes we will talk about as well. You can learn the basic heart rate, heart rhythm, and morphology of the deflections; you can also look for evidence of ischemia or infarction with this test.
- **Stress ECG**. This is also called an exercise ECG. Electrodes are placed on the patient, who then exercises on a treadmill or stationary bike to look for evidence of ischemia stress on the heart during exercise.
- **Ambulatory ECG**. This is done with just a few electrodes placed on the chest. The person is ambulatory for up to a week (depending on the test) to look mainly for evidence of ectopy that wouldn't necessarily be seen on the patient over a short period of time. These types of tests won't really check for ischemia in any reliable way, however.

You can also rely on telemetry, which is basically an ambulatory ECG using chest electrodes, often used in a hospital setting to track the patient's heart rate and rhythm remotely.

5-Lead Wire System

The 5-lead wire system is sometimes used when you want to put a person on "the monitor," or if you are entertaining a telemetry system. It helps you get valuable rhythm information plus some ability to look for ischemia. It often requires using a telemetry box attached to adhesive pads through short wires.

These are the electrodes you'll place:

- **Electrode 1**—on the right in the midportion of the clavicle (white electrode)
- **Electrode 2**—on the left side beneath the clavicle (black)
- **Electrode 3**—in the 4th intercostal space just right of the sternum (brown)
- **Electrode 4**—on the right side on the lowest part of the ribcage (green)
- **Electrode 5**—on the left side on the lowest part of the ribcage (red)

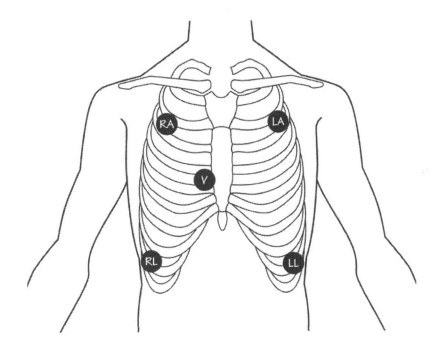

As you can see, the four corners form the four limb leads, and the brown lead in the middle forms the single precordial lead.

3-Lead Wire System

The 3-lead wire system is even simpler. You end up with three electrodes that collectively make for three leads, called RA, LA and LL. These are often used for ambulatory readings, to look for evidence of ectopy, or abnormal runs of tachycardia or bradycardia you won't get in a shorter reading. The electrodes are placed as shown:

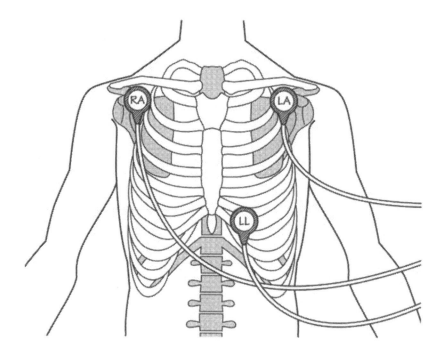

RA - **RED** electrode placed under right clavicle
near right shoulder within the rib cage frame.

LA - **YELLOW** electrode placed under left clavicle
near left shoulder within the rib cage frame.

LL - **GREEN** electrode placed on the left side below
pectoral muscles lower edge of left rib cage.

While the 3-lead system is good for detecting arrhythmias, it is not a good way to look for evidence of ischemia. This is because there is no precordial lead, so it is a 2-dimensional lead system that doesn't help you see what's happening along the heart's anterior wall. If you do see any ST-segment abnormalities, you should proceed in getting a 12-lead ECG.

Telemetry Systems

Telemetry is nice in a hospital setting, when you want to get a rhythm strip on your patient continuously, but the patient is often ambulatory. It requires a small box the patient wears in his or her pocket and enough leads (usually 3 to 5) to detect the heart rhythm. The information is passed along remotely so that someone at a distance can monitor the patient in real time.

The main thing you'll get is a beat-to-beat analysis of the heart during the collection time period. The box will store the data until the device is in range, should the patient become lost to remote monitoring for a period of time. It can also allow the patient to record any events they feel and what their symptoms were, to see if they are correlated. Some will have automatic triggers if there are arrhythmias, such as atrial fibrillation, bradycardia, pauses or tachycardia.

An Actual ECG Examined

The first thing you should know about ECGs is that the deflection on the tracing will be positive or negative, with regard to the vector or lead the segment of the ECG is recording. For example, if you are looking at any lead on an ECG, look to see if the deflection is positive or negative. If it is positive, its axis points toward the tip of the "arrow" or the vector's positive side, while negative is the opposite. It looks like this:

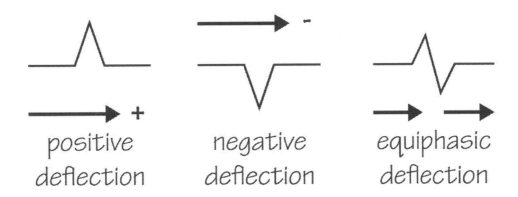

In equiphasic deflections, you will have both a positive and equally negative deflection. This is sometimes a judgment call when looking at an ECG tracing.

If you are doing a 12-lead ECG, you will get this page as your result:

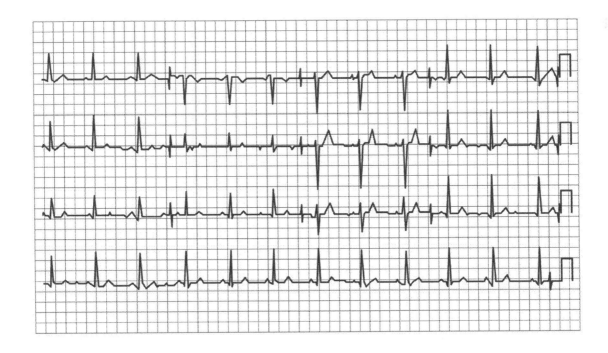

Pay attention to the order of the strips. There are four columns and three rows, appearing in this specific order every time:

I	aVR	V1	V4
II	aVL	V2	V5
III	aVF	V3	V6

When you apply the issue of deflection to the axis, you will be looking at the QRS complex. You will generally get this sort of thing:

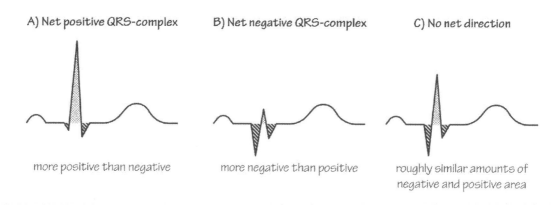

A) Net positive QRS-complex

more positive than negative

B) Net negative QRS-complex

more negative than positive

C) No net direction

roughly similar amounts of negative and positive area

You should note that this is truly a judgment call. First, find the baseline or isoelectric point. Estimate how much of the deflection is above or below the line. If you think most is above the line, call this positive and toward the vector's pointy end. If most of it is below the line, call it negative and toward the vector's non-pointy end. Sometimes it will truly be equal. Again, the vectors are in this direction:

Limb lead vectors:

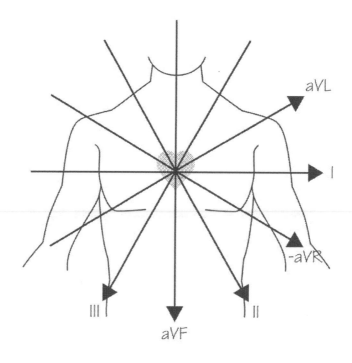

Precordial lead vectors:

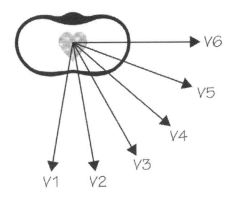

So far, we have only been talking about deflections specifically related to depolarization of the heart. The rules are different for repolarization. This table sums up the difference:

Depolarization	Toward the positive electrode	Positive Deflection
	Away from the positive electrode	Negative Deflection
Repolarization	Toward the positive electrode	Negative Deflection
	Away from the positive electrode	Positive Deflection

So what this means is that you can look at the specific leads and expect some obvious trends. For example, if the depolarization goes from the patient's right to left, this is the exact direction of the lead I vector, so the deflection will be positive. You would see minimal deflection in V1 and V2, which are perpendicular to lead I (and sticking out of the body in a forward direction).

Boxes and Sizes

We have talked about the grid you'll see on the ECG, but it's worth reviewing in detail now. There will be big boxes, and tiny boxes within them. The horizontal or x-axis is the time in the cardiac cycle; the vertical or y-axis is the voltage seen at the time. Each small box is 0.04 seconds (or 40 ms) horizontally and 0.1 millivolts vertically. Each large box is 0.2 seconds (or 200 ms) and 0.5 millivolts.

There is another feature you should think of as well, which is that the normal ventricle will deflect at a maximum height of about 10 millimeters or 1 millivolt. If you see it much higher than that, it is correct to suspect that there is some type of ventricular hypertrophy or enlargement in this patient. This is the grid and the reference height you should keep in mind:

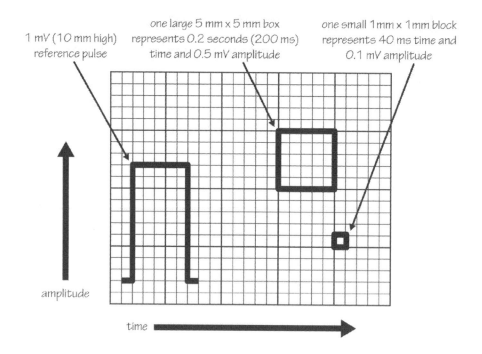

one large 5 mm x 5 mm box
represents 0.2 seconds (200 ms)
time and 0.5 mV amplitude

one small 1mm x 1mm block
represents 40 ms time and
0.1 mV amplitude

1 mV (10 mm high)
reference pulse

amplitude

time

Calibration

Conventional wisdom (and most user manuals) will tell you that ECG machines should be calibrated every six months or so, but you should do it anytime you suspect the reading you are getting is not correct.

The speed doesn't need to be calibrated, except to make sure it is set to run or "sweep" at 25 millimeters per second. The voltage, however, should be calibrated regularly. There should be a calibration button on the machine, which says "one millivolt" or "calibration," that will help you do this. After turning the machine on, press this button. You should see the square waveform shown below, and it should be exactly 10 millimeters in total height. This will calibrate the machine.

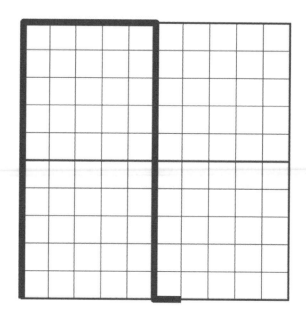

ECG Tools

Certainly, you can just "wing it" when looking at an ECG. When you get really good at reading them, you might be able to do it easily, but for now you should know that there are tools you can use to make a reasonable interpretation of what is going on. The height of the amplitude of any deflection is easy to determine, just by counting the boxes involved in the deflection and adding them up to get the millivolts (knowing that each box represents 0.1 millivolt). In the same way, you can simply add up the boxes between two horizontal points on the strip (like the R-to-R interval) to get the actual time elapsed (knowing that one big box [5 mm in width] is 200 ms, and therefore 5 big boxes is one second).

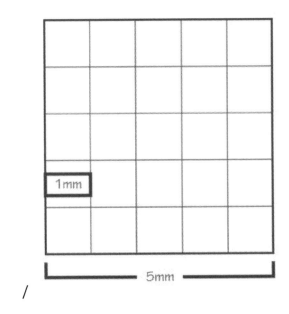

speed: 25 mm/sec

• 25mm = 1 second

• 5mm = 0.2 sec or 200 msec

• 1mm = 0.04 sec or 40 msec

There are a few ways to look at the heart rate simply by looking at the strip and not by reading the ECG interpretation given to you, including:

- **The Cardiac Ruler Method**. This is also called the "sequence method." You count the number of big boxes between consecutive R wave peaks. Each time you cross a big box from one to the other, say these numbers in order: 300, 150, 100, 75, 60, and 50. You can only do this if the rhythm is regular. It looks like this:

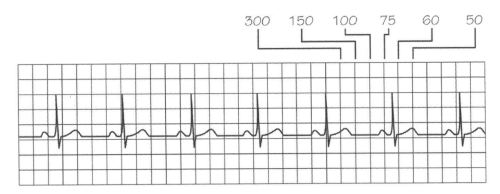

heart rate between 75 & 60 or ~ 70 / min

The heart rate in the above case is somewhere between 60 and 75 bpm, estimated at around 70.

- **The Six-Second Method**. You need to count thirty big boxes to get a total of six seconds of the tracing. Then count the number of R wave peaks you see in these six seconds. Multiply that number by 10 to get the heart rate. This works better for very slow rates or if the rhythm is not regular.
- **The Ten-Second Method**. This is even better for very slow rates. You count a longer stretch of big boxes, 50 total. Then take the number of R wave peaks in this stretch and multiply that by 6 to get your heart rate.
- **The 300 Method**. With this method, you take two R waves in a row and count the number of big boxes between these peaks. Take 300 and divide it by that number to get the heart rate. For example, if you count 5 big boxes between two successive beats, you take 300 and divide it by 5 to get a heart rate of 60.
- **The 1500 Method**—in this method, you count the number of tiny boxes between two successive R wave peaks. Then take 1500 and divide the number of boxes into this number to get the heart rate in beats per minute.

Calipers

You can also use a special caliper to measure an ECG, especially if you interpret ECGs frequently. This is what a typical one looks like:

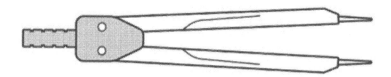

NOTE: A completely regular heart rate is generally not a good sign. A healthy or "more resilient" heart is not a metronome; instead, there is a natural variability to a normal heart called the beat to beat variability or the "inter-beat variability." These terms fit under the category of "heart rate variability"; a high variability level indicates a healthy heart.

The idea behind the calipers is to spread them out to match the R-to-R interval in two successive beats. Then keep the calipers the same in order to see if any or all of the other R-to-R intervals are the same as the one you first measured. Some heart rhythm disturbances will show progressively long R-to-R intervals. Diagnosing these arrhythmias is made much easier if you have calipers to help you.

Axis-Wheel Ruler

You can also get a basic ruler that has the axis key or wheel on it. It isn't used to measure the axis directly, but will remind you of what the axis you calculate actually means. The ruler looks something like this:

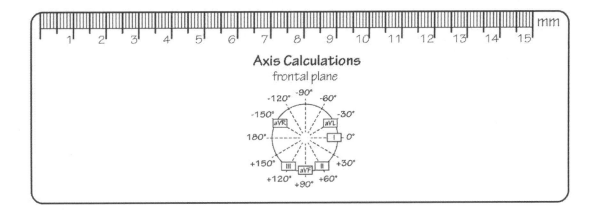

Axis Calculations
frontal plane

Accurately measuring the axis is typically not very important, but here's how you do it if you ever need to:

1. Look first at the standard 12-lead ECG and find the limb lead that is the most equiphasic (deflection the same above and below the isoelectric line).

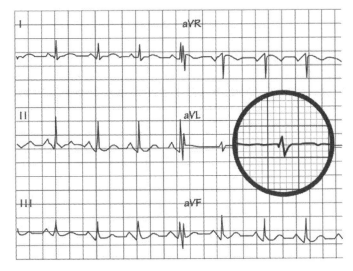

In this case, you can see that it is aVL that is the most equiphasic. Remember where this is on the wheel:

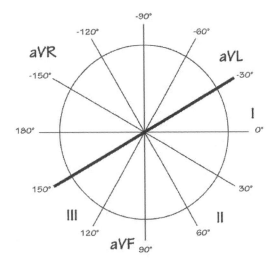

2. Now find the lead most perpendicular to this one. You can see that it is lead II.

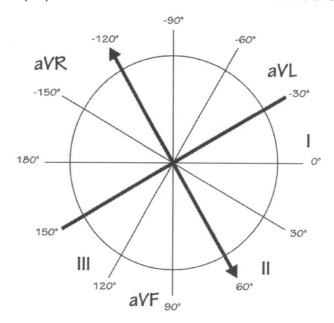

Look at lead II on the same strip to see if the deflection is mostly positive or mostly negative:

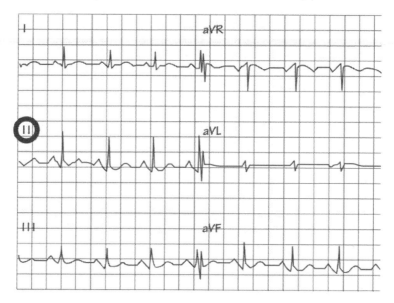

As you can see, it is mostly positive. The positive direction of lead II sits directly at 60 degrees. This means that the patient's axis is 60 degrees.

There is an online heart axis calculator you can also use to get an even more precise measurement of the axis (if that sort of thing is important in your situation). You have to look at the leads between the ones you are interested in, and measure the total height of the QRS complex in those leads.

To do this, you measure the height of the deflection above the isoelectric line in millimeters (make this a positive number); then subtract the height of the deflection below the isoelectric line (make this a negative number). It looks like this:

Lead I (for example) is + 12 millimeters based on this image:

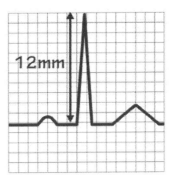

Lead III (for example) is +1 millimeter based on this image:

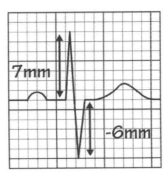

You would then plug those numbers into the calculator to reveal that the cardiac axis is 34 degrees, and therefore normal. It's super simple to use just those two leads to get a picture of the axis exactly.

You can use your ruler as a simple straight edge too. Why have a straight edge? It's because you want to know if things like the ST segment is depressed or not, and if the isoelectric line on the tracing is straight. You don't have to use anything fancy; just any straight-edged item, like a ruler, will do.

Obtaining a 12-Lead ECG

You already learned a lot about how to do a 12-lead ECG when we talked about lead placement. These 12-lead ECGs will give you a complete image of what's happening in the heart in clinical practice. It is the single most effective tool you have in looking for evidence of strain on the heart muscle, including whether or not the patient is having a heart attack. This would be the major reason to do this ECG versus any other type of simpler ECG technique.

Here are some tips for getting a good reading:

- Make sure there are no smartphones, tablets, or other electronic devices on or near the patient. These things will interfere with the ECG tracing by causing electrical interference and artifacts on the tracing.
- The patient should be supine or up to a semi-Fowler's position. This means that the head of the bed is at 30-45 degrees from the horizontal. If neither of these is possible, you can try sitting the patient up further.
- Have the patient lie with their arms at their side, shoulders relaxed, and legs straight (not at all crossed). Resting the arms across the abdomen will also work if the patient is too tense.

- Remind the patient that they should lie still and remain as calm as possible through the whole test.

If you see too much artifact, look for these possible causes:

- Electronic devices are present (remove them or shut them off).
- Cable loops are too close to a metal object (remove the cable loops from the metallic object, including the railings of the patient's bed).
- The electricity is surging (use a surge protector if this isn't already on the ECG machine).
- The cables or wires are cracked (inspect all of these to ensure they are all intact).
- The cables are not snuggly attached to the ECG machine (ensure the patient cables and the ECG device are securely attached).

Sadly for some of your patients, you will need to prep their skin. This means you will have to shave some men's hairy chests (and maybe some women's chests as well). Remove all oils and moisture from the patient's skin. You can accomplish this using an alcohol swab just over the areas where the electrodes will be placed. Ensure the environment is warm, so the patient is comfortable but not so hot that they continue to sweat.

Place the electrodes exactly as you've already learned to do to have the correct leads generated. The gel on the electrodes should be fresh and moist to the touch. If you don't get good contact with the moist gel, the signal will be inadequate. Use the same brand of electrode on the entire patient; don't mix and match. Avoid putting them over bones, and try to stay away from skin that has a major incision on it or that is raw or irritated.

Once you've got the patient prepped and the electrodes on, the ECG machine should be ready to deliver the reading. You will often be able to get a preview before you decide it's an adequate tracing. Within seconds, you will have your 12-ECG tracing completely ready for interpretation!

Interpreting a 12-Lead ECG

The ECG you get represents just ten seconds of your patient's life. It will not usually be enough to evaluate intermittent arrhythmias, but it will say a lot about any sustained rhythm and whether or not there is stress on the heart. A complete 12-lead ECG will show a few seconds (2.5 seconds to be exact) of each strip in the order we talked about already. You know now about the boxes and what they mean. You will also see a rhythm strip along the bottom of one or more leads, stretched out for the entire ten seconds. Here is an example of a good reading:

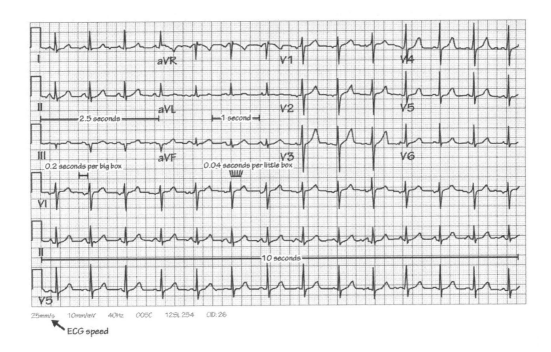

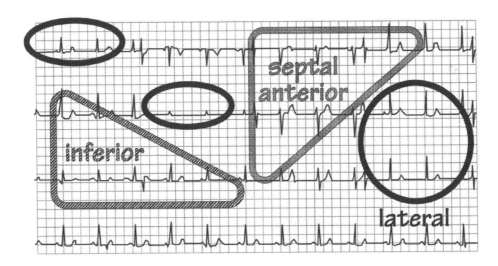

You should also be aware of the part of the heart most corresponding to each "section" of the 12-lead ECG, including the inferior, lateral, and septal/anterior parts. This rough drawing indicates where you would assess which part of the heart is involved in ischemia or infarction.

Now for some concrete steps as to what your interpretation should look like. You should try to get an overall look at it for a few seconds before diving in.

1. **Look at the heart rate.** In a normal ECG, the heart rate should be between 60 and 100 bpm if the sinoatrial node has anything to do with it. In children, of course, the rate will be higher than that. Anything below 60 bpm is "bradycardia," and anything faster than 100 is "tachycardia." You should use the QRS complex to determine the heart rate, even if the atria (p wave deflections) and the ventricles (QRS deflections) are not in sync with one another. We will talk a great deal later about the different issues you'll see in a "too fast" or "too slow" heart

rate, but for now you should know that the heart can still be abnormal even if the calculated rate is within normal limits. Use the tools you already know to get this heart rate established.

2. **Look at the heart rhythm.** We will talk a lot about abnormal rhythms soon, but you should be certain you can recognize what "normal sinus rhythm" looks like for now. Here's how you know you've got it:

   Look for a regular pattern of p waves and another regular pattern of QRS complexes. Make sure the P waves are the same in each lead and that the interval between the P wave and the QRS complex is the same throughout the ECG. Remember that this is the PR interval. In other words, look for this basic pattern:

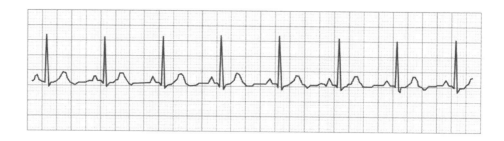

   Notice how you've got P waves and QRS complexes. Both are relatively regular, and each P wave is followed by a QRS complex at the expected time. We will talk later about measuring the PR interval and what it means to have a normal one. The QRS complex should look spiky and narrow; they should look the same in any lead you are looking at, but won't look the same from lead to lead. If you don't see this, you aren't dealing with normal sinus rhythm, so you'll have to figure out from there what you have (which we'll examine in more detail later).

3. **Find out what the axis is.** You already know how to determine this value. You can get at least a "ballpark" figure, which is helpful and most of the time the most detailed you ever need to get. If you need a particularly specific axis value, you know how to do this too.
4. **Look for evidence of something "not right" about it.** There are too many things that could be "not right" about an ECG to mention now, but you should be aware right away that you might see many possible things indicating the ECG isn't normal. Examples of abnormalities to look for are ST-segment depression or elevation, the presence of U waves, ectopic beats, wide variations in the beat-to-beat variability, and inverted or otherwise "abnormal" T waves. Again, the list is long, and you will be learning more as we dive further in later.
5. **Make your conclusions.** Once you do these things, sum them up with a statement that looks something like this (provided the ECG is normal): "This is a 12-lead ECG showing normal sinus rhythm with a heart rate of 65 beats per minute. The axis is normal at 60 degrees, and there is no evidence of ectopy or another arrhythmia present."

To Sum Things Up

The ECG is a great way to study the heart's electrical activity, using electrodes placed on the skin in places that can be far from the heart itself. You can pick up these electrical impulses because the human body has a great deal of saltwater in it, which conducts electricity nicely.

The electrodes are placed on the skin, but as you now know, these are not the "leads" you've maybe heard people call them. Leads are essentially electrical vectors generated by comparing the electrical impulses you get from one electrode to another. There are physical limb leads: three augmented leads (based on a virtual electrode theoretically located on the abdomen) and six precordial leads (generated from the chest electrodes you placed).

There are many different types of ECG you now know about, including resting ECGs, ambulatory ECGs, and stress or exercise ECGs. These are used for different purposes. Among the resting ECGs, you now know there are 3-lead ECGs, 5-lead ECGs, and 12-lead ECGs (plus several specialized ECGs used by cardiologists or researchers).

The 12-lead ECG is the best and most widely available tool for obtaining valuable information on the heart and heart muscle activity. You know how to obtain one and the things you need to look for. The basics you want to know include:

- What is the heart rate?
- What rhythm am I looking at?
- What is the axis?
- Is there anything else that just doesn't look right?

You hopefully now have the tools you need to make a basic 12-lead ECG interpretation. Now we will dig deeper into the different parts of the ECG deflections to prepare you for what you need to know to fully answer that last question: Is there anything that doesn't look right?

CHAPTER 3:
ECG COMPLEX

Even the best ECG interpreters often look only at the big picture when analyzing, including P waves, QRS complexes, T waves, and U waves. They also look at rate, the general pattern of rhythm, and probably the ST segment. This is enough most of the time. Still, a lot can be missed by failing to look at the ECG complex carefully. There are many pearls of wisdom you can uncover from studying these features.

Let's take some time now to separate each part of a single ECG complex. Each has a particular meaning you will understand more clearly by the end of the chapter. We will talk a bit about certain pathological conditions you will be able to detect after studying the ECG waves. Even though we have not gotten into them very much yet, you will be able to use the chapter as a reference later on, as you study the different heart issues that can be detected on an ECG.

Depolarization and Repolarization Reviewed

First, let's review exactly what you are looking at on an ECG. You are looking at defections, movements of the ECG tracing both above and below the isoelectric point. In this case, you are looking specifically at the electrical impulses on the body surface that have traveled or "propagated" to each site through the saltwater in your body.

Imagine you had a segment of the heart muscle depolarizing from the left side to the right side in a bath of saltwater. It would look like this:

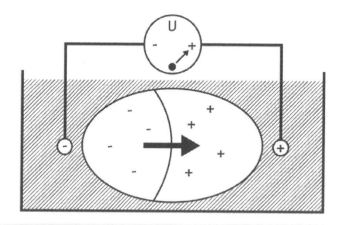

The cells at rest would be positive on the outside and negative on the inside. When the cells on the left depolarize, the cell becomes negative on the outside instead. The muscle cells on the right are still positive, so the lead on that side (if there was one) would be positive. This would mean that a positive deflection on the ECG at that time would be seen in that lead. Afterward, if all cells are now negative, you would see a zero reading on a meter (or no deflection on the ECG).

Remember, this is a dynamic process. Depolarization spreads over time, so the ECG tracing (which is sweeping across the monitor or page) will show a dynamic rise and fall in the tracing you see.

Any time you see a positive deflection, the lead you are looking at has more cells with positivity on the lead's positive vector side. In other words, if you are looking at lead I (positively pointing to the patient's left-hand side), it will show a positive deflection as the depolarization wave spreads from the patient's right to his left. It looks like this:

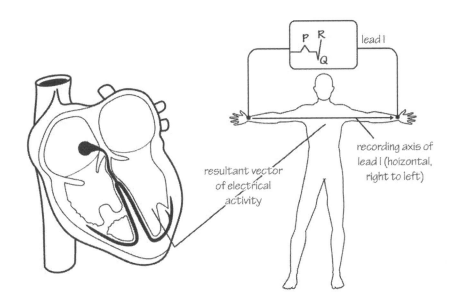

Repolarization involves going from a net positive charge outside the cells to a net negative charge. It will start at the spot that depolarized first, and spreads in the same direction it first depolarized. This will lead to a negative deflection on the same lead's tracing until all the cells have repolarized. The deflection will then go back down to zero.

The atria repolarize from the SA node first, which is where the whole process starts before spreading to the rest of the atrial cells. This doesn't mean much practically, because you don't see this repolarization on the ECG. It is hidden in the QRS complex.

The ventricles are different. The last cells to depolarize will be the very first cells to repolarize again. This means that for ventricular repolarization, you will get a positive deflection as these ventricular cells repolarize. The height of the repolarization depends on the mass of the tissue, so thicker walls in any of the chambers will lead to a higher repolarization peak.

The P Wave

Based on a typical cardiac cycle, the first thing that must happen in order to start the process is the depolarization of the SA node in the right atrium. This spreads across its entirety, as well as the left atrium. It is almost always a positive deflection on the ECG strip. A normal p wave is less than three of the small squares, or less than 0.12 seconds.

Look for a smooth ride up and a smooth ride down. In lead II, I will always be monophasic, but in lead V1 it will always be biphasic. Monophasic means it is like a hill, going up and then down; biphasic is like a hill and valley, first going up above and then down below the isoelectric point, then back up to baseline. You will see this:

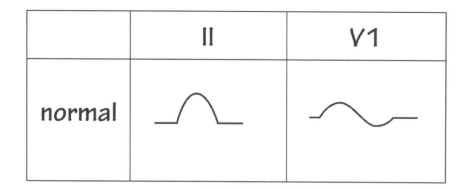

	II	V1
normal		

In aVR, it will be inverted (a valley without a hill). This is because its positive direction is mostly to the right (opposite in many ways to lead II). It has an axis that is maximal at zero to around 75 degrees. Look for an amplitude of about 2.5 mm in the limb leads, or 1.5 mm in the precordial leads. The p wave is most prominent in the limb leads II, III, and aVF, or in the V1 lead; if it shows an abnormality, it will be in these leads.

Because the SA node is in the right atrium, this will depolarize first. The p wave you see below is a combined effort from both atria, but it is a divided p wave. The first third is all the right atrium; the last third is all the left atrium. The middle third is made from a combination of both atria:

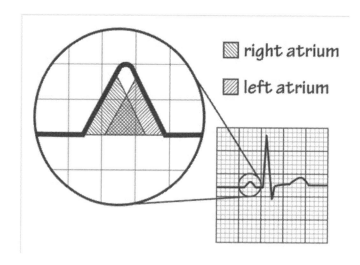

right atrium

left atrium

Because of where V1 sits, the right and left atriums depolarize in opposite directions (from that perspective only). This leads to the biphasic pattern you see on this lead. The upward deflection is the right atrium, and the downward is the left. This is important because it will help you decide if one atrium is enlarged but the other is not.

The P Wave in Lead II

So what if the right atrium is enlarged? In lead II (which is where you should look for this), you will see a lopsided higher peaked p wave. The right atrium is larger, so the depolarization lasts longer than it should. This depolarization peak slopes over onto the left atrial component, so the total wave will be taller even though the width is still less than 0.12 seconds. It looks like this:

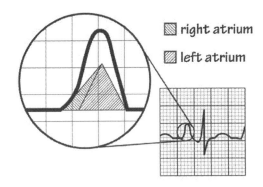

If the left atrium is instead enlarged, this depolarization time will be longer. The p wave height you get won't be bigger, because it doesn't slop over onto the right atrial part of the p wave. Instead, it lengthens the p wave. You might even see a notch at the top, which is called "p mitrale" if you see it. It looks like this:

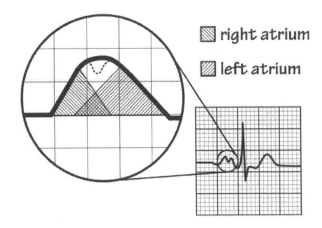

The P Wave in V1

If you aren't sure if there is an atrial enlargement in lead II, then confirm your suspicions in lead V1. Remember, it is biphasic. If the right atrium is enlarged, the positive deflection will be greater than 1.5 mm. You need to measure its height from the isoelectric line to the peak of the hill.

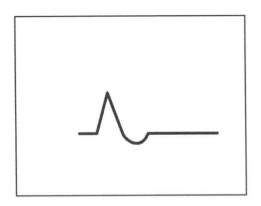

If the left atrium is instead enlarged, the downward deflection of the p wave is larger (or deeper) than it should be. If you measure the p wavelength, you'll see that it will often be greater than 40 ms wide. The depth will be greater than 1 mm. It will look something like this:

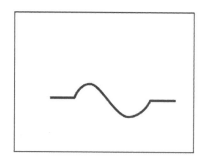

If both atria are enlarged, you will see something of a mixed effect. In lead II, look for notching and a wider p wave than normal. In lead V1, look for a wide and unusual-looking p wave. They often look like this:

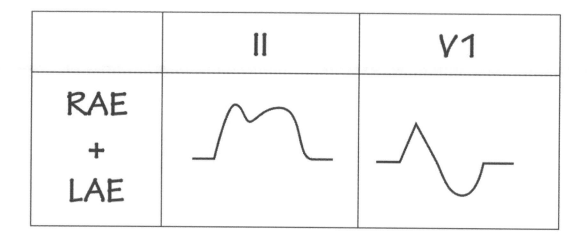

Other P Wave Findings

You can see now that the p wave will tell you a lot about what is going on with the atria. It will actually tell you even more than this, however, including:

- **P Mitrale**. This is also called having bifid p waves. You will see this if the left atrium is enlarged, and it might have you think of mitral valve stenosis. Some other causes of P Mitrale are mitral valve regurgitation, hypertension, and hypertrophic cardiomyopathy. This is because for any cardiac disorder where the outflow of the left atrium will be blocked, the increased pressure behind the valve enlarges the atrium. It looks like this:

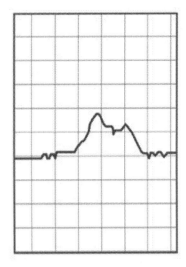

- **P Pulmonale**. This is what you'll see if the right atrium is enlarged. The p waves will look peaked, as the middle is the sum of the enlarged right atrium and the normal left atrium.

  Note the high, peaked shape of the p wave in this situation. This is seen in certain lung diseases where there is pulmonary hypertension. Imagine the extra pressure in the lungs preventing the smooth flow of blood from the heart's right side. This would naturally cause high pressure on the right side of the heart, including the left atrium. Other disease processes where you may see this include chronic obstructive pulmonary disease (COPD) and acute pulmonary emboli.

- **Inverted P waves**. These are seen in ectopic atrial rhythms. This means that the rhythm originates outside of the sinus node. One such rhythm is a junctional rhythm s (when the heartbeat is first triggered by the AV node instead of the SA node). The p wave is inverted because the depolarization is essentially backward. It looks like this:

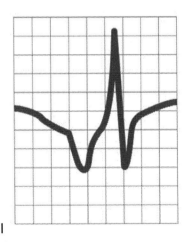

The p wave is mostly inverted in the lower or "inferior" leads. If you see the PR interval normal at less than 120 ms, the AV node is the source of the abnormal beat causing this problem. If the PR interval is long at more than 120 ms, the ectopic beat comes from somewhere inside the atrium.

While the SA node is the main driver of the heartbeat, there are other sources in the heart that can generate an extra beat. An extra beat in the atrium is called a PAC or premature atrial beat. It is always premature (early) because it needs to be. If it were not, the SA node would kick in before it could happen.

- **P Waves with Different Shapes.** This is called variable p wave morphology. It means that there are different areas of the atrium randomly contributing their own heartbeat. This will lead to a p wave that looks different all the time. Some people will have palpitations, but not everyone. It looks like this:

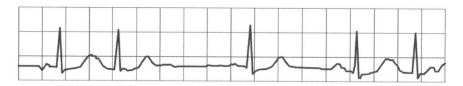

If the heart rate is too fast (greater than 100 bpm) and you see at least three different p wave shapes, it is called multifocal atrial tachycardia.

The PR segment and interval

The PR interval and the PR segment are actually two different things, as seen below:

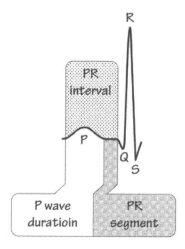

As you can see, the PR interval is the time between the beginning of the P wave to the start of the QRS complex.

Did you know? Despite the name, the PR interval does not go to the start of the R wave as you would think, but to the start of any deflection at all in the QRS complex. For example, the start of the QRS complex can often be a downward deflection, known as a "Q wave." In that case, count the PR interval from the start of the P wave to the start of this Q wave, even though it isn't actually the R wave at all.

The PR interval is the time it takes for the electricity to get to the AV node. It should be about 120 to 200 ms, about 3 to 5 small squares on the standard ECG. If it is longer than that, it is called a first-degree AV heart block.

If the PR interval is less than expected or less than 120 ms, this is called a pre-excitation syndrome. It means that there is some abnormal pathway in the atrium that is sending the beat faster to the AV node than normal, causing the ventricles to contract too early. It can also mean that the beat is starting at the AV node instead of the SA node. The p wave will be inverted, or you might not even see any P wave at all. Junctional rhythms look like this:

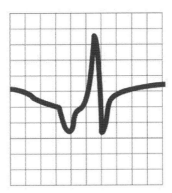

We will talk a lot about AV blocks in another chapter, but briefly, there are four of them you should know about as they relate to the PR interval. As mentioned, a PR interval longer than 200 ms means that an AV block exists, and that the electricity took too long to get processed through the AV node.

A first-degree AV block is seen when the PR interval is long but consistently the same length. Count the boxes; if you see more than 5, this is a first degree AV block. It looks like this:

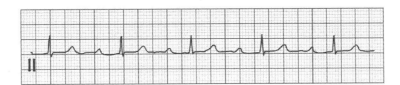

Notice how long and consistent this interval is?

If you don't see consistency in the PR interval's length, you should look at other types of blocks as well. Second-degree blocks come in two types, called Mobitz I and II. Mobitz I involves a prolonged PR interval that doesn't stay the same. The first isn't very long at all, then they get progressively longer, until one P wave is blocked from transmitting a QRS complex at all. This will happen only once, then will start the same pattern over again, like this:

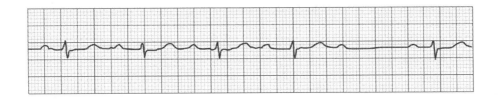

Mobitz II looks different. The PR interval can be normal or prolonged. The key feature here, though, is that some P waves are completely dropped. You call this one a 4:1 block, because it takes 4 p waves to get the QRS complex. In the case shown below, there is a hidden one inside the P wave after the

QRS complex because of the T wave that is already there. You know this because the P waves are regular and the QRS waves are regular, but their regularity doesn't match. You have to assume the P wave you can't see is there because it is predicted to be there.

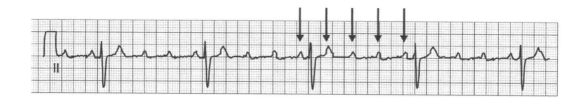

Did you know? *Woldemar Mobitz was a German internist who lived from 1889-1951. He observed these patterns of arrhythmia representing some kind of heart block, and knew they were distinct from each other. In 1924, he published his work on these, which were later called Mobitz type I (or Wenckebach) and Mobitz type II (or Hay). Interestingly, he had a hard time finding work, because he had chronic tuberculosis of the throat, and people thought he was contagious.*

Third-degree AV block happens when there are P waves and QRS complexes, but they have no relationship to one another. The P waves will be faster, but as they don't even affect the ventricles, the QRS waves happen by themselves, often at a much slower rate. It looks like this:

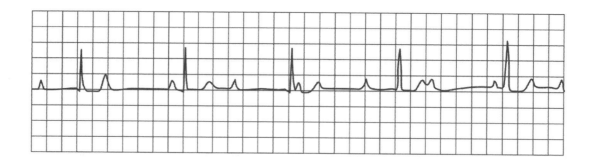

There are two pre-excitation syndromes with shortened PR intervals, called Wolff-Parkinson-White syndrome and Lown-Ganong-Levine syndrome. Both of these have accessory pathways, not the normal one from the SA node to the AV node. These are faster, which explains the shorter PR interval.

This accessory pathway is actually a reentry circuit, like a loop you'd put on your favorite song, doing the same pathway over and over again. Again, they need to be faster than the normal SA node pathway to override it.

Wolff-Parkinson-White syndrome is a short PR interval problem, with a wide QRS complex containing an odd upstroke called the delta wave. It looks like this:

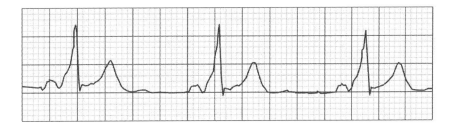

See that strange pattern of the QRS complex? It's wide, and it has a slow upstroke before it speeds up to a normal height. This is what makes the QRS complex so wide. In Wolff-Parkinson-White syndrome, there is essentially an extra electrical pathway between the atria and the ventricles, which will lead to a rapid heartbeat. This syndrome is considered relatively rare and is present since birth.

With Lown-Ganong-Levine syndrome, the PR interval will be short—often very short. The QRS complex is normal, and there are no delta waves. The patient will report feeling tachycardia. It looks a lot like this:

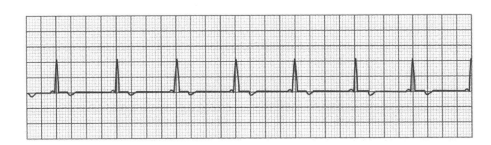

The PR Segment

The PR segment is the time period from the end of the P wave to the start of the QRS complex. You will find this to be important in situations of atrial ischemia and pericarditis. In cases of acute pericarditis, the PR segment will be depressed, along with a strange saddle shape to the ST segment, which will also be elevated except in aVR and V1, where it will be depressed. It looks like this:

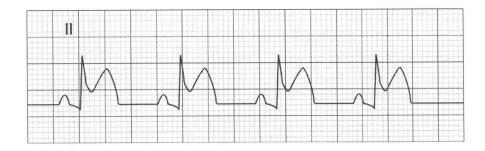

In atrial ischemia, the PR segment will be either depressed or elevated. This is seen if the person has had a myocardial infarction involving the atria. People who have this finding have a poor prognosis in general, because it means they have a higher risk for certain rhythm disturbances and rupture of the heart wall during the recovery period. This is what PR segment depression looks like:

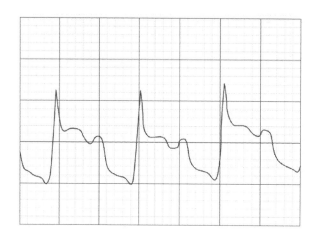

The QRS Complex

As you know, the QRS complex is the representation of ventricular depolarization. Both the height and width of this complex are important to pay attention to. The shape of the complex is also important, as it will say a lot about what is happening in these two chambers.

Notice that we always say QRS, even when there isn't always a Q, R, and S wave visible. If you need to get picky about it, you can call specific waves in the QRS complex by the specific names you see here:

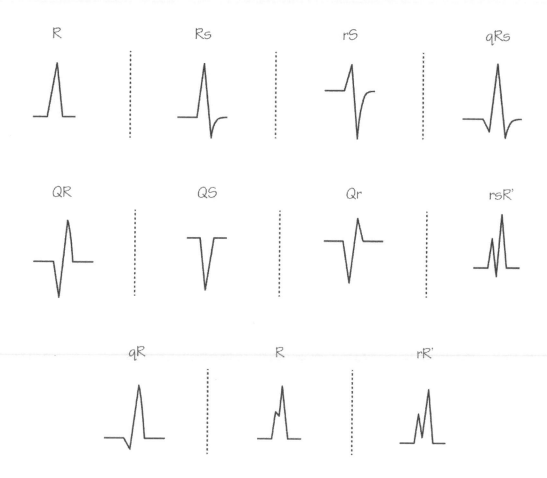

If a wave is tiny, it is called by its lower-case letter. If it is big, it is called by its upper-case letter.

The width of a normal QRS complex is between 70 and 100 ms. If it is less than 100, you should think of a supraventricular origin in the atria. If you see a QRS complex wider than normal, you should think of a ventricular origin, or what's called ***aberrant conduction*** of electricity in the supraventricular area. Here we see an ECG with both normal and widened QRS complexes:

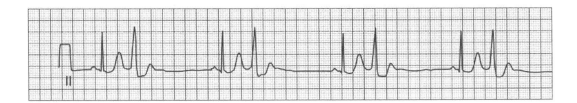

Narrow QRS Complexes

The three main rhythms are seen when the complex is narrow: normal sinus rhythm, atrial flutter, and junctional tachycardia. You will find a narrow QRS complex in one of three different states:

- The P wave comes from the SA node and will be normal.
- The P wave comes from somewhere else in the atria. This will be an abnormal P wave, often seen in atrial flutter.
- The wave starts near the AV node (also called the junction). You won't see a P wave at all, or you will see some type of abnormal P wave and a short PR interval.

Let's look at these rhythms more closely, one by one.

Normal sinus rhythm is a regular rate pattern with a heart rate of 60 to 100 bpm, seen in a healthy person. There are normal p waves and a narrow QRS complex, usually with a small Q wave, and R and S waves that look different depending on the lead. This is what it looks like:

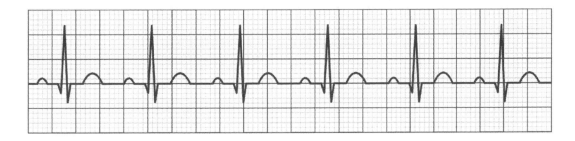

Atrial flutter is rarely a healthy pattern, but the QRS complex will be narrow. A focus of electricity is generated in the atrium (not usually the SA node, however). The rate of atrial beats is usually so fast that the QRS complex cannot keep up. You will see this in the sawtooth pattern of P waves, some of which are buried in the QRS complex. Every third P wave is linked to a QRS complex in this picture, but this complex will still be narrow as you can see.

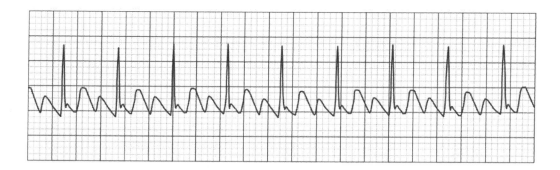

Junctional tachycardia is a fast rhythm (note the "tachycardia" in the name). The origin of the beat is in or near the AV node. Regardless, it must actually go through the AV node for the complex to be narrow. The P wave will be upside down or right-side up, depending on the lead. It will look something like this:

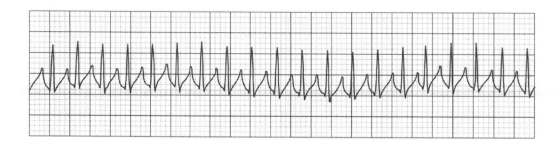

Wide QRS Complexes

An abnormal QRS complex is anything greater than 100 ms. Still, it takes a QRS complex greater than 120 ms to get a true rhythm from the ventricle, or a bundle branch block (where one of the bundles to a ventricle is damaged or delayed). There are a lot of reasons to have a wide QRS complex, including:

- Any bundle branch block
- High potassium levels (hyperkalemia)
- Tricyclic antidepressant overdose or other sodium-channel blocking toxins
- Pre-excitation disorders like WPW (Wolff-Parkinson-White syndrome)
- Using a ventricular pacemaker
- Having hypothermia
- Any type of intermittent aberrancy (usually related to the heart rate)

Let's look at the different types you might see. In ventricular tachycardia, the heart rate is fast and coming from the ventricles. You won't see any P waves at all. As you can see, the heart rate is very high. As you can imagine, this is a bad rhythm to have, because it often degenerates further into ventricular fibrillation (often a kiss of death for those who have it). Ventricular tachycardia or VTach looks like this:

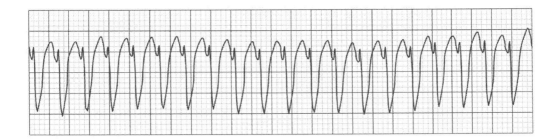

It can be tough sometimes to determine if the rhythm is ventricular or supraventricular. This is because the QRS can be wide in supraventricular tachycardia if the electricity travels in an unusual path. One way to check if this is VTach and not SVT (supraventricular tachycardia) is to look for these things:

- No evidence of left or right bundle branch block
- An extreme axis deviation (to the patient's upper right side)
- Complexes longer than 160 ms
- If there are P waves, they are at a different rate than the QRS complexes
- There might be some beats where the SA node captures the rhythm to produce a normal sinus beat randomly
- You might see fusion beat, which is a combination of QRS complexes and another deflection
- You will see all precordial leads with QRS complexes positive or negative entirely
- RSR-prime is seen, which is an R wave plus another R' wave that is taller on the left than on the right (very specific for VTach)

You will see some of these features here. The C is a captured beat, and the F is a fusion beat:

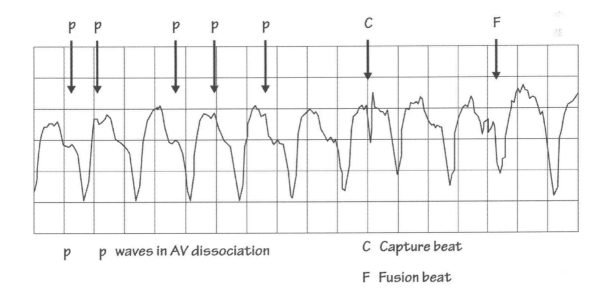

p   p waves in AV dissociation   C Capture beat

F Fusion beat

SVT with aberrancy of the electrical conduction should be suspected if you see these things:

- The person is young and has no heart disease
- The person has a known bundle branch block

- The person has a known history of SVT that has been treated with known successful SVT treatments.

SVT with aberrancy can look like this:

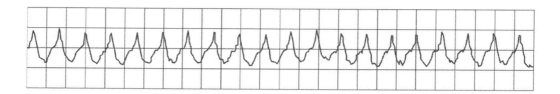

It can be tough to tell the difference, so doctors often have to guess and treat, to see what works to resolve the rhythm abnormality. There is an algorithm that can help decide what the rhythm is. You have to follow it from the top to the bottom to get your answer:

Brugada Algorithm

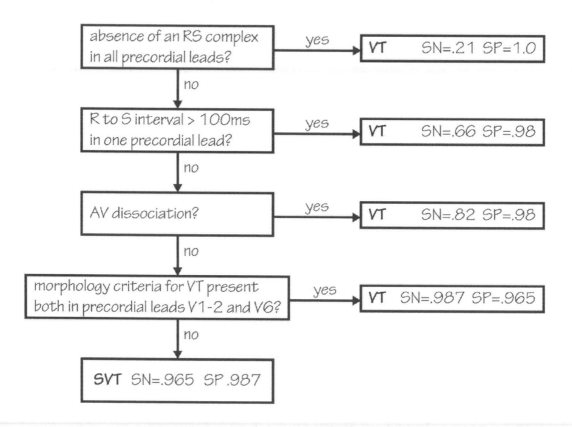

Did you know? Two Spanish brothers—both physicians—are credited for identifying Brugada syndrome in 1992. Pedro and Joseph Brugada discovered some unusual ECG patterns in people who suffered from sudden cardiac death. Since discovered, we've learned the syndrome is genetic, so people are born with it but don't have symptoms (fainting, palpitations, or sudden heart-related death) until they reach their 30s or 40s.

Other things to notice that can help lead you to decide what type of pattern you are looking at (all having a wide QRS complex) include:

- **Right bundle branch block (RBBB).** You will see an RSR' wave in V1, and really deep and unusual S waves in the lateral (left-sided) leads.
- **Left bundle branch block (LBBB).** You will see an S wave dominance, especially in V1. The R waves will be wide without seeing Q waves in the lateral leads.
- **Hyperkalemia (high potassium levels).** Look for other things, such as very peaked T waves.
- **Tricyclic antidepressant toxicity.** Look for a rapid sinus rhythm, plus a tall R-prime wave seen in the aVR lead.
- **WPW (Wolff-Parkinson-White syndrome).** Look for the short PR interval, plus the delta waves you've already seen.
- **Ventricular pacing.** You will see these pacing spikes that don't look like they belong with any type of ECG tracing. They look like this:

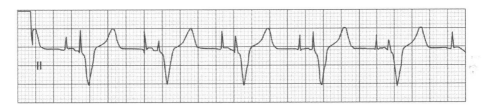

- **Hypothermia.** This is a situation where the heart rate will be very slow and the QT interval will be long. Shivering can cause a lot of artifact. You will see an Osborn wave as well, which is a large dome-shaped wave after the QRS complex. Exactly what this is has not been fully established. Take a look at this observed pattern:

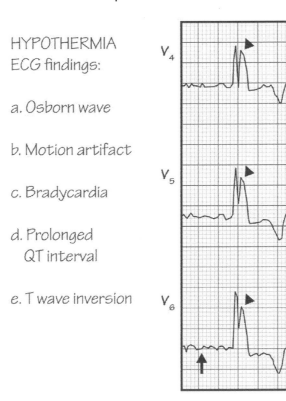

HYPOTHERMIA ECG findings:

a. Osborn wave

b. Motion artifact

c. Bradycardia

d. Prolonged QT interval

e. T wave inversion

High and Low Voltage QRS Pattens

In most cases, the QRS is elevated if the left ventricle is particularly enlarged (known as left ventricular hypertrophy). It could be a normal finding in a young athlete, however, or a very slim person. Exactly how you define "high voltage" depends on who you ask.

The most commonly used method for defining a high voltage QRS complex is the Sokolov-Lyon criteria. A QRS complex is called "high voltage" if there is an S wave in V1 and any R wave height in V5 to V6 (whichever is highest) that add up to more than 35 mm total. If you see QRS complexes that are too tall, don't automatically think of left ventricular hypertrophy unless you see other evidence of it (more on that later). It looks like this:

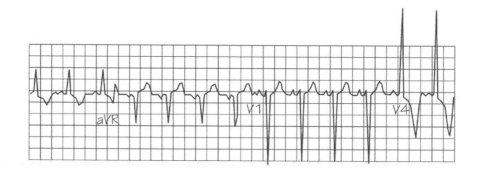

If the QRS height is too low, you might see these things: 1) the total QRS height in the limb leads is less than 5 mm, or 2) the total QRS height in the precordial leads are less than 10 mm.

Electrical alternans is an ECG finding showing a QRS complex that is different in height each time. This is often seen when a huge amount of fluid is in the pericardial sac. The heart sloshes around in it, so the QRS complex appears different over time. It looks like this:

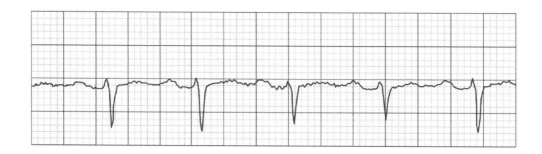

Notched QRS and Prime Waves

The QRS complex will sometimes be strange-looking for a wide variety of reasons. The different patterns you might see include:

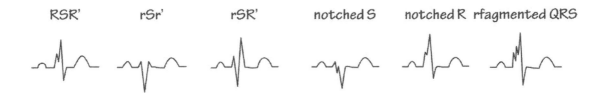

RSR'   rSr'   rSR'   notched S   notched R   rfagmented QRS

These are often seen in situations where the myocardium has some kind of scar on it, for example a myocardial infarction. Others are seen with left ventricular hypertrophy plus some kind of conduction defect to the ventricles.

Specialists can look at the specifics by using special filters that eliminate stray electrical activity and artifacts. These really narrow down what the irregular or fragmented QRS complex is coming from. Though a fragmented QRS complex is interesting, it takes a super-specialist to actually figure the whole thing out. This is what one looks like:

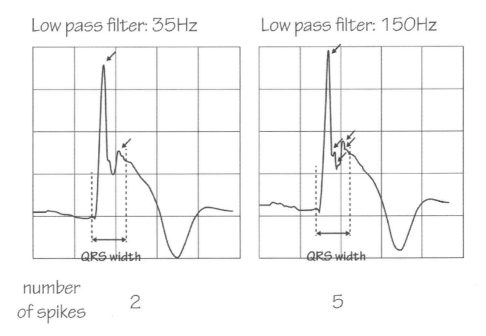

Low pass filter: 35Hz   Low pass filter: 150Hz

QRS width   QRS width

number of spikes   2   5

See how much more information you get by filtering out the artifacts and looking at the QRS complex very closely. Again, you shouldn't be expected to figure it all out, even if you see one of these. The causes are often scars, however.

Q Wave

The Q wave is any initial downward deflection on the QRS complex. The key here is "initial" because it has to be before the R wave. It is the representation of a tiny left-to-right-sided depolarization of the interventricular septum. You will see a small one on the left side of the patient for the most part (as in leads I, aVL, and V5 to V6). It looks like this:

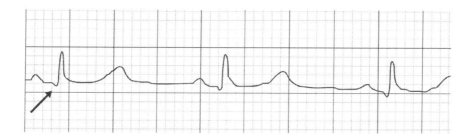

Most of the time, you will see small Q waves as normal findings in practically all leads. If they are deeper than 2 millimeters, they will also be normal in lead III and lead aVR. On the other hand, the Q wave shouldn't be seen on the right-sided precordial leads (as in leads V1 through V3).

When is a Q wave considered "abnormal"? Situations include:

- A widened Q wave of greater than 40 ms or one box wide
- A Q wave deeper than 2 mm if in any other lead than II and aVR
- More than 25 percent of the total depth of the entire QRS complex is made of the Q wave part
- Anytime you see a Q wave in leads V1 through leads V3

Most abnormal Q waves indicate a past heart attack but not a current one. Certain less common disorders that might lead to a pathological Q wave are extreme rotations of the heart, infiltrative diseases of the heart muscle, and hypertrophic cardiomyopathy. If you didn't place your leads right, you would also see "pathological" Q waves.

Is it abnormal to have no Q waves, even when you should see one normally? Yes—in fact, it can be a problem. If you don't see Q waves in V5 and V6, you should suspect a left bundle branch block.

See these big Q waves in the inferior leads (lead III and aVF)? This would clearly indicate a probably inferior myocardial infarction (a heart attack along the bottom of the heart):

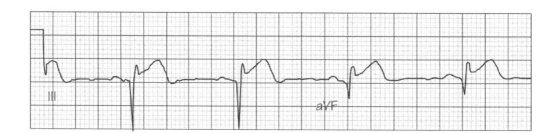

This ECG would show a giant anterior MI because you see Q waves in these precordial leads:

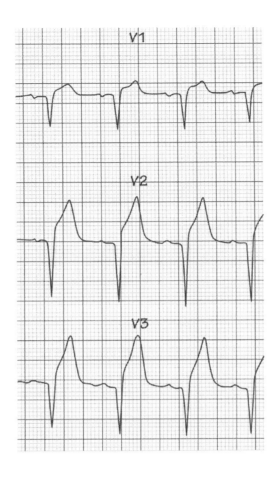

The ST segment

The ST segment is the normally flat line near the isoelectric line between the end of the QRS complex to the end of the T wave. It looks like this:

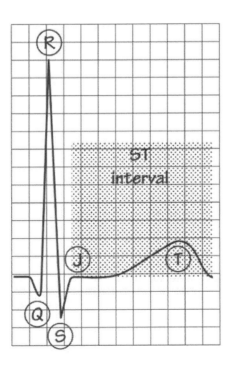

It represents the time frame between ventricular depolarization and when it repolarizes again. This is an important segment to look at because it will say a lot about whether there is myocardial ischemia or true infarction. The term "ischemia" means the heart is suffering from low oxygen levels, and the tissue is dying. The term "infarction" means that a section of the heart is dead. In contrast to the Q wave, you will see the ST segment changes almost immediately after an event to the heart has happened.

ST-Segment Elevation

While a lot of ST-segment elevation usually means a heart attack is happening, it doesn't have to mean this. There are about a dozen other possibilities you have to consider by looking at the patient's history and symptoms. They include:

- Spasm of the coronary arteries (Prinzmetal's Angina)
- Pericarditis
- Left bundle branch block
- A benign condition where the ventricles repolarize early
- Ventricular aneurysm
- Brugada syndrome
- Any pacemaker activity on the ventricles
- Takotsubo cardiomyopathy (broken heart syndrome)
- High levels of pressure inside the brain
- Left ventricular hypertrophy

You can actually get widely different appearances when the ST segment is elevated. Here are some examples:

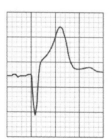 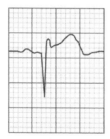 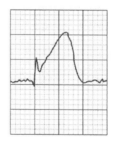 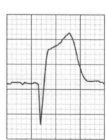

With ECGs, the patterns of the ST-segment elevation mean everything. You will see the ST-segment elevation vary according to where the heart attack is located. For example, these are the patterns that mean the most:

- Septal heart attack, seen most in lead V1 and V2
- Anterior heart attack, seen most in V3 and V4
- Anterior septal heart attack, seen in V1, V2, V3, and V4
- Lateral heart attack, seen most in leads I, aVL, and leads V5 and V6
- Inferior heart attack, seen in leads II, III, and aVF
- Right ventricular heart attack, seen in leads V1 and V4 (if placed on the right side of the patient)

- Posterior heart attack, seen in posterior leads not often used, like V7 and V9

Look too for confirmation by checking leads that are electrical "opposites" of one another. If an elevation is seen in leads I and aVL, check for depression in lead III.

There is no true infarction in coronary vasospasm, or what's called Prinzmetal's angina, but spasm in the coronary arteries. The ST segment will be elevated but only when the individual is having chest pain at the time of the ECG. You will be able to tell the difference if the patient gets better on their own or if vasodilators are given to open up the vessels.

Pericarditis is basically obvious if you know what you're looking for. The ST-segment elevation will be widespread and involve a saddleback appearance of this segment. You will often see PR segment depression as well. A few leads will show a reciprocal or opposite ST-segment depression in some leads (especially in aVR or V1). It can look like this:

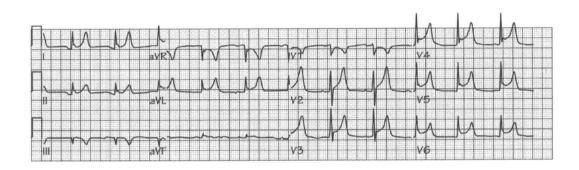

A concrete sign seen almost exclusively in pericarditis is called Spodick's sign, identified in 1974 by David Spodick. It's a downward sloping of the TP segment, which is supposed to be relatively straight. It is best noted in leads II and the lateral precordial leads. See this example:

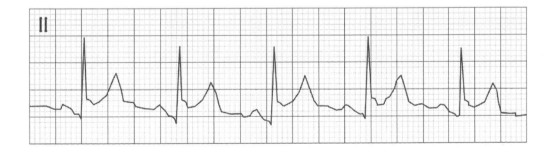

If the ST-segment elevation is benign and just due to early repolarization, the elevation will be minor, and the T waves will be particularly tall. The J point, a sharp demarcation point between the QRS and the isoelectric line, will look like a fish hook. It is usually more prominent when the heart rate is slower. It can look like this:

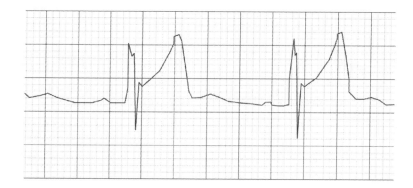

A left bundle branch block or LBBB involves ST-segment elevation opposite to what you'll see in the QRS complex. If the QRS complex lies mostly below the isoelectric point, the ST segment will be elevated. On the other hand, if you see the main body of the QRS above the line, the ST segment will be depressed. The T wave will be the same way. It looks like this:

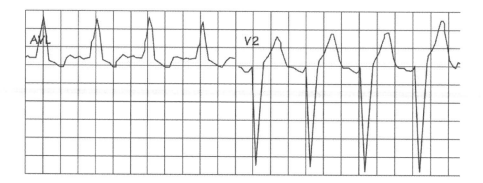

In the example shown, the left-hand side mostly has an upright deflection of the QRS complex, and the ST segment/T wave is below the line. On the right-hand side, the QRS complex's deflection is mainly below the line, so the ST segment is elevated, and the T wave is upright.

Left ventricular hypertrophy is similar to an LBBB; the ST segment is elevated in those leads with deeper S waves (especially in V1 through V3). The opposite is true with those having high R waves. Because this involves ventricular hypertrophy, you can expect the QRS complexes to be too tall as well.

A ventricular aneurysm involves ST-segment elevation with deep Q waves, mostly because an aneurysm is a side effect of having an older heart attack. It comes on because of the scarring there, plus the fact that the aneurysm will move out when the rest of the heart is contracting and moving inward. It can look like this:

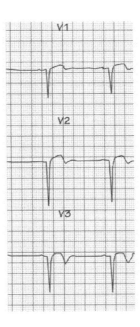

In this case, you'd expect to see an anteroseptal MI with the aneurysm being in that region because the ST segment is very elevated in leads V1 through V3.

Brugada syndrome can be seen in the standard ECG. It shows up as ST-segment elevation and a partial right bundle branch block or RBBB seen mainly in V1 and V2. It looks like this:

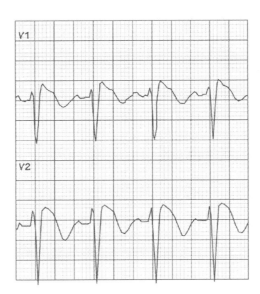

So why does increased intracranial pressure in the brain cause ST-segment elevation? It isn't because the heart is ischemic or that there is pericarditis. No one knows for sure, but it's thought to be due to either stunning of the heart wall itself, or because of the increased levels of epinephrine and norepinephrine in the bloodstream after the event.

The T waves will often be depressed and very elongated or wide. These are called cerebral T waves because they are seen so often in these cases. Look especially for these findings:

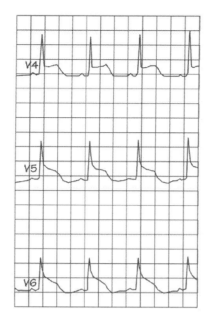

See how the ST segment is elevated, but goes directly from the elevated ST segment to the upside-down T wave, so that you see a vague sloping pattern.

Takotsubo cardiomyopathy often shows ST-segment elevation as well. You might see that a real heart attack has taken place at some point, but this isn't a given. The T waves might also be inverted in a person with an ECG showing this disorder.

Did you know? Takotsubo cardiomyopathy is also called "broken heart syndrome." This is because it is seen when a person really does have an emotionally broken heart. It isn't named after any scientist named Takotsubo, though, but rather a Japanese fisherman's octopus-trapping pot (tako meaning "octopus" and tsubo meaning "pot"). It probably would be stressful to be an octopus in such a pot. A Japanese scientist called Sato identified it in 1991, and it is caused by stunning of the myocardium by a rush of adrenaline during stress.

Less commonly, you might see ST-segment elevation in cases like these:

- Acute pulmonary embolism
- High potassium levels
- Dissection of the aortic wall
- Drugs that block the sodium channels
- The heart converting to a normal sinus rhythm
- High blood calcium levels
- Low body temperature

Like anything in ECG analysis, it can be tough to make a clear-cut decision about what is wrong with the patient without the benefit of some type of history and physical examination.

The ST segment can be depressed as well. You should think of these things when looking at a depressed segment:

- Ischemia of the myocardium
- Effects of digoxin
- Low potassium levels
- Right bundle branch block
- Right ventricular hypertrophy
- Supraventricular tachycardia (SVT)
- LBBB
- Left ventricular hypertrophy (LVH)
- Any ventricular paced rhythm

The T Wave

The T wave will usually be a positive deflection seen after every QRS complex. It must be there if the ventricle has depolarized, because it has to repolarize after that. This is what the T wave represents. The TP interval is the time period after the T wave is over but just before the next P wave has begun again. It will be upright in every lead except for aVR and lead V1. It should be less than 5 mm in height in the limb leads and less than 10 mm in the precordial leads. They should be shorter in general among women. The QT interval is measured (not the T wave interval itself) when looking to see if the duration is too long.

There are a lot of kinds of abnormalities you might see, including:

- **Peaked T waves**. This is seen especially in hyperkalemia (high potassium levels). These are what they look like:

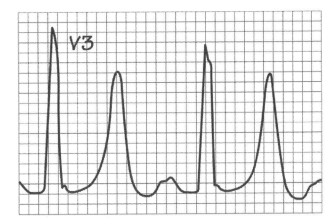

See how hard it is to tell the difference between the R wave and the very peaked T wave?

- **Hyperacute T waves**. These are broad and kind of peaked. They might show up first in an MI and will be seen before the ST segment actually rises. It might look like this:

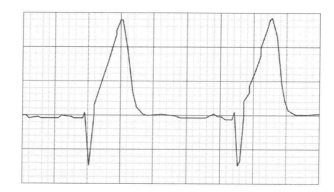

- **Inverted or upside-down T waves**. Can be normal in children and can be seen in a heart attack. Any bundle branch block can show inverted T waves, and you'll see them if the left ventricle muscle is too thick. Other possibilities for inverted T waves are hypertrophic cardiomyopathy, pulmonary embolism, and high intracranial pressure. Expect it to be inverted in lead III. If you have an old ECG to look at, you should call it abnormal if the T wave inversion seems new. Deep T waves that are inverted more than 3 mm are more likely to be abnormal.

- **Biphasic T waves**. These are T waves that flip from rightside-up to upside-down. Look for them in cases of low potassium levels or an ongoing heart attack with ischemia of heart muscle. An UP first, then DOWN second T wave is seen in myocardial ischemia, while the reverse is true for low potassium or "hypokalemia." These look like this:

myocardial ischemia   hypokalemia

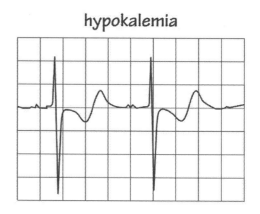

- **"Camel hump" T waves**. These are double-peaked T waves that look like a camel's back. These really aren't double-peaked waves from the ventricle, but are either U waves stacked on an existing T wave, or P waves hidden in the T waves themselves. This is seen in heart block cases where the P wave is not marching at the same rate as the QRS complex and matching T wave. A prominent Q wave situation looks like this:

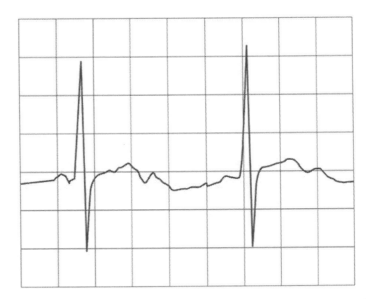

- **Flat T waves** (although not completely flat, certainly). These don't necessarily mean something bad, but can indicate situations where the myocardial ischemia is early in the course of the disease or mild. It can also mean that the patient's potassium is low. This is what you'll see in some hypokalemia cases:

More on T Wave Inversion

If this is a situation of myocardial ischemia or infarction, the leads where you see the inversion is important. If the heart is stressed in the organ's inferior part, you will see the inversions in leads II, III, and aVF. If the MI is lateral, look for inverted T waves in leads I and aVL, and precordial leads V5 and V6. If the MI is in the heart's anterior part, look for abnormal T waves in leads V2 through V6.

Here's where context is important. If the T wave changes over time (dynamic), you should think more that it represents ischemia. If the T waves are inverted and stay that way, the problem is more likely to be an infarction (permanent myocardial cell death).

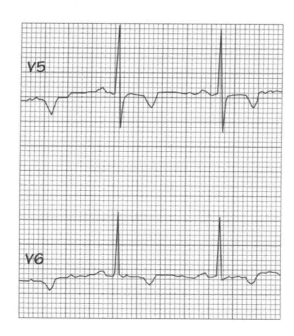

In left ventricular hypertrophy, the T wave will often be inverted in those leads that shouldn't normally be inverted. You will see the high amplitudes in the QRS complex, as we've talked about. It can look like this:

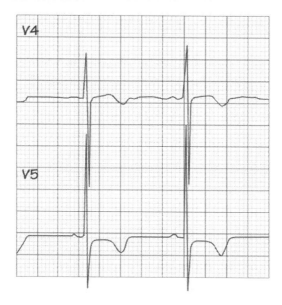

When you see T wave abnormalities, like inverted T waves where they shouldn't be, you need to think of strain on the heart. This is why it is sometimes included and defined as a "strain pattern." In cases of pulmonary embolism (blood clots in the lungs), the right ventricle will be strained by pushing blood out to blood vessels that aren't open or patent. In such cases, the T wave will be inverted mainly in leads V1 through V3 and the inferior leads (II, III, and aVF).

The U wave

The U wave is not seen in most normal ECGs. They are small, less than 0.5 millimeters in total deflection, and occur in the same deflection direction as the T wave they follow. They are most prominent in leads V2 and V3. There are different theories as to what causes it, although likely repolarization of the ventricle's Purkinje fibers, or perhaps a prolongation of repolarization of certain cells in the myocardium called "M cells." It's also possible that it is from mechanical forces placed on the ventricular wall itself.

Another feature of a normal U wave is that it will be more prominent if the heart rate is very slow. If it is below 65 bpm and you can see them, it is probably normal. Expect it to be less than a quarter of the corresponding T wave's total height next to it. Any larger than that are likely to be abnormal in some way. This is a normal one:

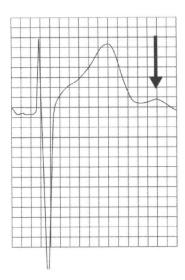

Abnormal U waves are either too prominent or inverted. Let's look at prominent U wave first:

All U waves higher than about 2 mm or more than 25 percent of the T wave height are abnormal. It would help if you thought of these as possible causes of:

- Very slow heart rates
- Severely low potassium levels
- Low calcium levels
- Low magnesium levels
- Low body temperature/hypothermia
- Hypertrophic cardiomyopathy
- High levels of intracranial pressure
- Left ventricular hypertrophy
- Digoxin use
- Use of certain antiarrhythmic drugs
- Use of drugs for psychosis called phenothiazines

Expect to see long QT intervals if the U wave is prominent. These go together often.

This is a case of more prominent U waves because the heart rate is prolonged:

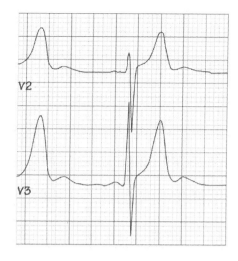

These are U waves seen with low potassium levels:

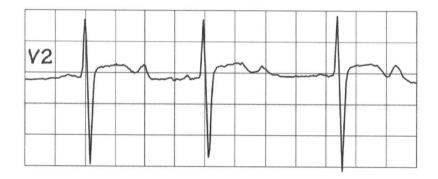

U Waves That are Inverted

Anytime the T wave is in one direction (usually upright), but the U wave is in the other (usually down), this is abnormal. Any negative deflection of a U wave should be very suspicious for some type of heart disease. Common causes of an inverted U wave include:

- Ischemic heart disease
- Valvular heart disease
- High blood pressure
- Congenital heart disease
- Hyperthyroidism
- Cardiomyopathy

Again, context is important. The person with inverted U waves who also has chest pain should be considered as having myocardial ischemia until proven otherwise. This is an early marker for things like unstable angina and early myocardial infarction. In fact, you can assume that the LAD (left anterior descending artery) is probably more than 75 percent blocked somewhere. You can see this here, for example:

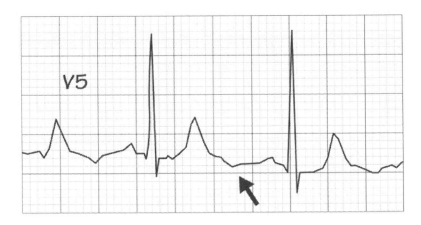

The QT interval

The QT interval is from the start of the Q wave to the end of the T wave. It is the entirety of ventricular depolarization and repolarization. You can see this time frame here:

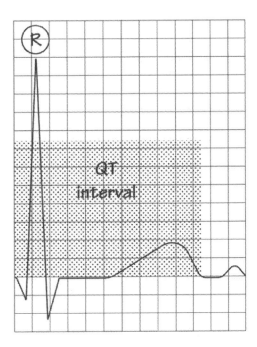

These are the rules for what you will see concerning this segment on the ECG strip:

- The QT interval will shorten if the heart rate is fast and lengthen if the heart rate is slow.
- A long QT is not a good sign because it will increase the chances of ventricular arrhythmias.
- On the other hand, the QT interval can be too short due to genetics. These people have an increased chance of developing VFib, paroxysmal atrial fibrillation, and sudden death from a rhythm disturbance.

You should try to measure the QT interval. Do it in any of these three leads: V5, V6, or lead II. Measure several beats and then take the maximum as being the answer. You should see the U wave, but only if it is fused with the T wave (you have to do some creative geometry at times). Don't include those that aren't merged. This is what you need to do if the U wave is merged with the T wave:

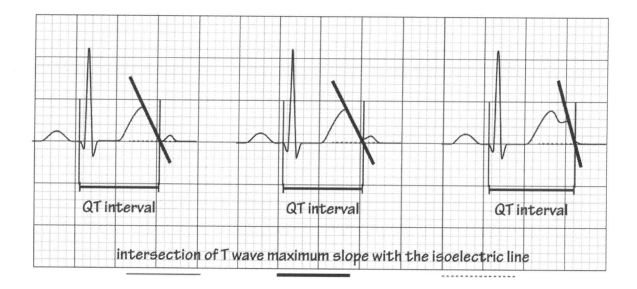

QT interval   QT interval   QT interval

intersection of T wave maximum slope with the isoelectric line

There is such a thing as the "corrected QT interval." It is calculated at any heart rate but is standardized to determine if the heart rate was 60 bpm. It is a better way to see if the patient's QT interval is a problem or not. Multiple formulas are used to get this normalized number. You don't need to memorize these, mostly because the ECG machine might be able to get that number for you through its own internal calculations. There are even free phone apps that will calculate this for you.

If the QTc (the normalized version) is longer than 440 ms in men or 460 in women, this is prolonged. Any number greater than 500 ms increases the chances of developing an abnormal ventricular arrhythmia called Torsades de Pointes. If the QTc is shorter than 350 ms, this is too short.

There are a lot of reasons to have a long QT interval, including:

- Low potassium
- Low magnesium
- Cold patient
- Low calcium
- Myocardial ischemia
- High levels of intracranial pressure
- Congenital diseases
- Resuscitation after a cardiac arrest
- Certain medications

This is what you'll see if the potassium is too low. It doesn't always look obvious, so you need to measure it directly:

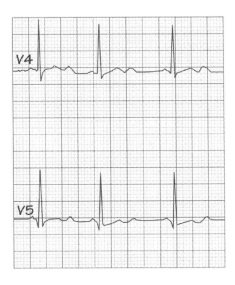

There are U waves in this image, so you have to include its length as well. The QTc is about 500 ms here, especially seen in the precordial leads. You will see the same thing with low calcium or low magnesium, so these might have to be measured to see the cause of this problem.

A short QT syndrome (or short QTc) can be due to high calcium levels, the effects of digoxin, or congenital short QT syndrome. This is what you might see if the calcium levels are too high:

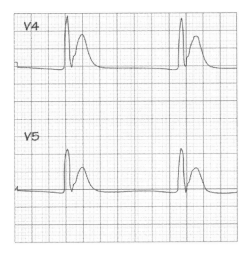

See how the T wave comes right after the QRS complex in this image? It is visibly "too short" if you've looked at these kinds of things a lot.

Congenital short QT syndrome is an autosomal dominant heart disease, where the heart's potassium channels are abnormal. The result is a QT interval of fewer than 280 ms. The T waves are often very tall and peaked. The QT interval doesn't get much better when the heart rate slows down. This is what you'll see:

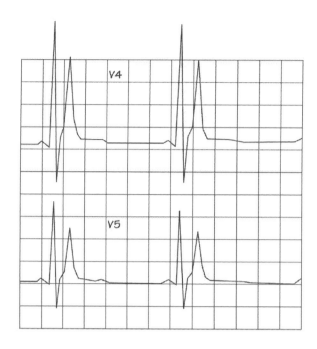

Suspect this syndrome if you see these things in a patient's history or physical exam:

- A young person who develops atrial fibrillation
- A known family member who has this syndrome
- Someone in the family who had sudden cardiac death at a young age
- A QTc of less than 350 ms and very tall and peaked T waves
- No difference in the QT interval with changes in heart rate

You can use a nomogram on any rhythm strip to see a person's risk of developing the potentially lethal Torsades de Pointes (or TdP). When you see the nomogram here, you should know that if the patient's QT interval is above the nomogram line, the risk exists of developing TdP. These people need to be monitored very carefully.

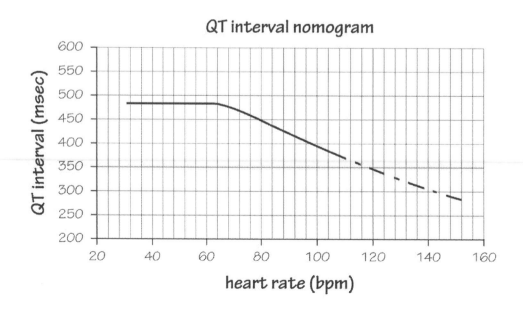

To Sum Things Up

Now you know that ECG tracing is far from a simple squiggly line. Each deflection up or down means something potentially significant about the person's health. You should consider each lead carefully and note when you expect the deflections to look a certain way. You should know the relationship between what you'll see in one lead versus another. If the leads weren't placed right, you should be able to figure that out.

This chapter talked a lot about different rhythm disturbances without really explaining them carefully. These will be covered in the next chapter. Still, you can look at a specific QRS complex and dissect its meaning now. This should help you understand why you see the things you can see during certain rhythm disturbances.

CHAPTER 4:
ARRHYTHMIAS

The normal rhythm of the heart is called *normal sinus rhythm* or NSR. The electrical impulse originates from the SA node. You know now what it looks like: a P wave, the same PR interval each beat, a narrow QRS interval, a regular and normal QT interval, and a similar T wave for each beat. If you do not see this, you need to look for an arrhythmia and determine what kind it is. This chapter will talk about arrhythmias, what they look like, and where they come from. We will also talk about some treatments used for the different arrhythmias.

Clinical manifestations of arrhythmias

Arrhythmias can feel very different from one another; it is hard to pick one symptom and say that's what an arrhythmia feels like. Most people have felt an arrhythmia at least once. You might describe it as a "butterfly" in your chest or a fluttering sensation of some kind. Most of these are totally normal and do not mean you have heart disease. But there are other symptoms of an arrhythmia that are far more serious.

Not all arrhythmias are just skipped or extra beats here or there. Depending on how fast or slow your arrhythmia is, you might have more noticeable symptoms, most directly related to low cardiac output (low output from the ventricles). This is because the arrhythmia has made the heart inefficient. Common signs and symptoms include:

- Weakness or fatigue with exercise
- Lightheadedness, dizziness, or fainting spells
- The sensation of a rapid heartbeat
- Chest pain or pressure in the chest
- Sudden collapse or sudden cardiac death

It can be tough to determine the patient's arrhythmia; this is why it is important to get an ECG to see what's happening. Some rhythm disturbances are so transient that you won't catch them on a 12-lead ECG. Instead, you would need to use a Holter monitor or a Zio Patch, which is a single-lead patch that detects arrhythmias for 7 full days.

Causes of arrhythmias

There are so many possible causes of an arrhythmia, including heart damage that blocks a normal pathway in the heart, drugs or hormones that cause excitability in the heart's electrical system, or areas of excitability and abnormal pathways causing reentrant arrhythmias. You will see how these work in a moment.

These are the major causes of an arrhythmia:

- Anatomical changes in the heart (think of things like congenital heart diseases that prevent normal transmission of impulses in the heart)

- Reduced blood flow to areas of the heart (as in heart attacks or other areas of ischemia to the heart that don't involve a true heart attack)
- The restoration of blood flow after a procedure used to treat a heart attack in progress
- Scar tissue in the heart that prevents the normal flow of blood
- Exertion or strain that causes increased stress hormones (adrenaline) in the heart
- Excesses of thyroid hormone or reduced thyroid hormone, leading to rapid or slow heart rate respectively
- Low blood sugar causing premature beats or slow heart rate
- Electrolyte disturbances, mainly calcium, magnesium, or potassium
- Exertion or strain
- Conduction disorder, which directly affects the pathway of electricity in the heart
- A loss of a natural pacemaker (the sinus node), with an ectopic center elsewhere in the heart taking over

It isn't possible in all circumstances to figure out where an arrhythmia comes from by looking at the ECG, but there are telltale signs that you can use at times to have a good idea of what might be causing the disturbance.

Types of arrhythmias

Let's get a one-stop look at the different arrhythmias. We will talk a lot more about what these actually look like so you can see for yourself the signs to look for to recognize these easily. Remember to think about a rhythm disturbance as being primarily ventricular or atrial (supraventricular) in nature.

Bradycardia

If you encounter an average heart rate lower than 60 bpm, it is called "bradycardia." Most of these cases are sinus bradycardia, which means everything is normal except that the heart rate is initiated too slowly. It is seen in elderly patients and athletes. Athletes are bradycardic because their heart is so efficient from continual exercise they do not need to have it beat as frequently. In other cases, the sinus node is abnormal, so beats don't get generated as quickly.

Did you know? The slowest heart rate ever recorded in a healthy human belongs to Daniel Green, a UK athlete who happens to be 81 years old. His heart rate dropped to 26 beats per minute when he was formally tested. Many younger male athletes have similar heart rates in the 27-28 bpm range. Runners, cyclists, and rowers tend to have the lowest ever recorded heart rates.

Tachycardia

Any heart rate greater than 100 bpm is considered to be tachycardia. Most of these will be sinus tachycardia, often brought on by stress or exercise. Adrenaline (epinephrine) will stimulate the SA node to send out atrial signals faster than it's supposed to. Some tachycardias are abnormal, especially those that are too fast to support a normal cardiac output.

Ventricular Tachycardia

This is an often dangerous heart rhythm disturbance involving a heartbeat origin in the ventricles. As you can imagine, the QRS complex will be wide. Single ventricular beats or PVCs are not necessarily abnormal, but many of these in a row should raise a suspicion that this is not normal.

Ventricular Fibrillation

This is a rhythm disturbance you don't want to have. It is the most commonly recorded rhythm seen in a sudden cardiac arrest that is witnessed and recorded fast enough (before the heart stops and the person dies). There are multiple parts of the ventricles trying to fire at once. It is not compatible with consciousness because there is no real cardiac output. There are no QRS complexes or P waves that are recognizable or predictable. You can't fix this rhythm without defibrillating the heart or "shocking it." This will cause a pause or refractory period that you hope is resolved by having some normal part of the heart kick in to start a more normal rhythm.

Supraventricular Tachycardia

Supraventricular tachycardia or SVT involves a heartbeat starting in the atria. Caffeine, tobacco, alcohol and cold medications tend to cause these. Depending on the person, the heart rate can be nearly 200 bpm. Like elevated thyroid function and rheumatic heart diseases, some disorders can show up as SVT that might need treatment if the rhythm is persistent. Persistent SVT is also called PSVT or paroxysmal SVT.

Atrial Fibrillation

In this rhythm, the atria do not generate a rhythm; the QRS is narrow in general, but the P waves are absent. The main risk is for stroke, because the atria do not contract. The flow of blood is slow enough that blood clots can build up on the atrial wall. Miniature clots break off from an area of the left atrium; from there, they travel to the brain to cause an embolic stroke. Atrial fibrillation or AFib is the most common cause of stroke. We will talk about this in a moment.

Wolff-Parkinson-White Syndrome (WPW)

WPW is a fairly dangerous heart rhythm disturbance involving abnormal pathways between the atria and ventricles. The electrical signal gets to the ventricles sooner than expected, leading to a fast heart rate and frequent fainting. The rhythm is characteristic, as you will see. The same people prone to WPW also have a tendency toward having PSVT on other occasions.

Atrial Flutter

This is where the atria emit a high-speed heart rate and regular P waves one after the other. Most people's hearts cannot keep up with all of these P waves, so there is blockage of some of them, usually every 2-3 beats. The greater the P waves ratio to QRS complexes, the slower the actual ventricular rate will be. This rhythm is hard to sustain; it often degenerates into atrial fibrillation.

Heart Block

We have already talked about heart block and will talk about it in more detail in the next chapter. A summary of these phenomena is shown here:

- First-degree AV block. This is simply a prolonged PR interval.
- Second-degree AV block. This is where some P waves are dropped and not transmitted as QRS complexes. Mobitz I involves an orderly prolongation of PR interval until one is dropped. In contrast, Mobitz II involves dropping several P waves in a row and a slow ventricular rate.
- Third-degree AV block. This is a complete heart block and involves P waves and QRS complexes not connected to one another. The ventricular rate is prolonged in almost all cases.

Next let's dive more deeply, so you can see exactly what these look like. You should be able to identify them fairly easily on the ECG, although a few are hard to define at first glance.

Sinus node arrhythmias

If you have to have any arrhythmia, this is the one you want to have. It is also called "respiratory sinus arrhythmia," or RSA. It means the heart rate falls and rises with breathing, so it is not regular. The vagus nerve acts on the heart in variable ways depending on inhalation and exhalation, which is why you get RSA. Children have this normally, but the chances of having this are less in older age. If you see this, it signifies a resilient heart and a decreased chance of cardiac death.

This is what you'd see in RSA if you tracked breathing along with it. The heart rate increases with inhalation and decreases with exhalation.

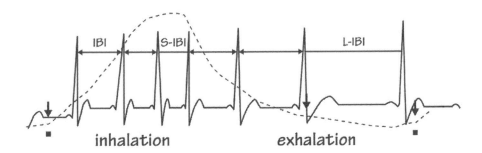

Sinus tachycardia

You should be able to recognize sinus tachycardia easily. The rate is greater than 100 bpm but not generally much higher than 150 at rest. The P waves and QRS complexes are normal, and the rate is regular. This is completely normal if you are exercising or are experiencing some type of stressor. If you see this, you need to decide if this is normal or temporary, versus a sign of early heart disease.

Temporary and compensatory reasons for sinus tachycardia are pain, anxiety, exercise and stress—anything that triggers a fight-or-flight response and an increase in adrenaline/epinephrine in the body. A more worrisome cause is early heart disease. Inflammation of the heart muscle, pulmonary embolism, cardiac tamponade, hypoxia, low blood sugars, dehydration, and electrolyte disturbances in the body cause stress on the heart, often leading to sinus tachycardia. Thyroid hormone in high amounts increases metabolism, so the heart must beat faster.

There are so many medications and illicit drugs that cause sinus tachycardia. Caffeine is the main culprit, but you also have to consider antihistamines, decongestants, and albuterol. Amphetamines and cocaine will do this as well. Even nicotine can increase the heart rate. Withdrawal from numerous drugs will also trigger sinus tachycardia. Think about withdrawal from benzodiazepines, alcohol, beta-blockers, and digitalis.

Sinus tachycardia is fairly easy to identify. The main thing you'll find is the rapid heart rate. Everything else in the ECG will be normal. This is not a rhythm you need to treat, although you might need to hunt for a cause and remove it to reduce the heart rate.

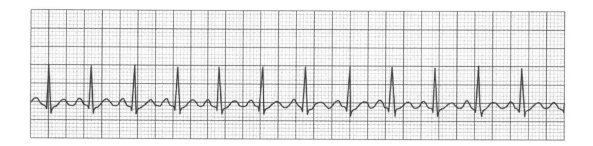

Sinus bradycardia

This is also an easy rhythm to identify. It looks like a normal sinus rhythm but much slower (below 60 bpm). Make sure to look at all the P waves to make sure each one goes on to cause a QRS complex. You should also make sure the PR interval is normal (0.12 - 0.20 seconds). As mentioned, it is normal in athletes.

There are many reasons why sinus bradycardia might be due to something much more serious than being physically fit. You might see it during or after a heart attack, after trauma to the chest, and in sick sinus syndrome, where the sinus node is damaged. Anything that inflames the heart, such as Lyme disease, rheumatic fever and myocarditis, will also potentially lead to sinus bradycardia.

Just as there are drugs that increase the heart rate, there are those that decrease it. Beta-blockers, digoxin, lithium, opioids, cannabinoids, and calcium channel blockers will do this. Other blood pressure medications will do this too. Stimulating the vagus nerve (as when a patient needs to be suctioned) will trigger transient bradycardia. People with low thyroid function are at risk for bradycardia. The same is true for those with anorexia, high potassium levels, sleep apnea, and anything causing low oxygen levels (hypoxia).

It will look essentially normal with expected P waves, QRS complexes, and PR intervals when you see this. You will want to look for any possible dangerous causes of this and fix those.

Few drugs provide long-lasting relief from symptomatic bradycardia. Atropine will briefly speed up the heart, but if you want something that lasts longer, you should instead consider having the person evaluated for a permanent pacemaker. Pacing the heart is the best way to speed it up, by sending a signal for it to contract faster than the signal coming from the heart's pacemaker itself:

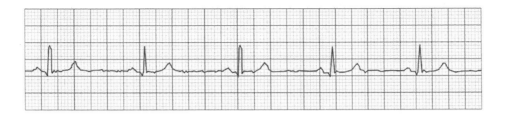

Most of the time, sinus bradycardia is not serious. The exception is sick sinus syndrome. If this isn't treated promptly, only about half of these people live another five years.

Sinus arrest

It probably isn't healthy to have sinus arrest or sinoatrial arrest either. This is when the SA node just quits sending out a signal for a minimum of two seconds, even though it can last up to a couple of minutes. The good news is that the atria are filled with other pacemaker cells just itching to get in there and take over. These parts of the heart kick in after a few seconds, and the pace is reset (usually slower than the sinus node itself would be). It looks like this:

Sinus arrest

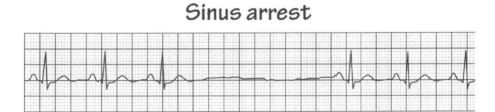

These extra beats cause what is known as an *escape rhythm* (maybe because the person escapes death when this happens). Atrial escape rhythms have a rate of 60-80 bpm while a junctional escape rhythm has a rate of about 40-60 bpm. The further down the electrical pathway you get, the slower the heart rate will be if that part sets the pace. Sinus arrest can also be paced using a pacemaker.

Sick sinus syndrome

Sick sinus syndrome or SND (sinus node dysfunction) is pretty much what it sounds like. The sinus node is not healthy and often sends signals out too slowly to the rest of the heart. It is possible for the heart rate to be too fast, or alternate between being too fast and too slow. This latter problem is called *Tachy-Brady syndrome*.

What would cause the sinus node to behave this way? There are two main reasons. The SA node could have scar tissue called fibrosis that causes it to send out poor signals to the heart. The second reason is extrinsic factors acting on an SA node that isn't too sick itself. In reality, most sick sinus syndrome is age-related. There are also hereditary reasons to have a damaged SA node.

Extrinsic causes of sick sinus syndrome usually affect the vagus nerve to the heart itself. Remember that the vagus nerve directs heart rate through the parasympathetic branch of the autonomic nervous system. This is called the vagal brake because it puts a brake on the SA node. In autonomic diseases or carotid sinus hypersensitivity, this is exaggerated at times. Also, many electrolyte disturbances can cause SA node slowing. These are the causes you should most consider:

- Hypokalemia
- Hyperkalemia
- Hypothyroidism
- Increased intracranial pressure
- Drugs or toxins
- Hypocalcemia
- Hypoxia
- Hypothermia
- Obstructive sleep apnea

The SA node is made of two types of cells. The P cells are the ones that set the pace, while the T cells propagate this electrical pacing to the rest of the heart. When these cells fail, bradycardia can be sudden and severe. You can also have sinus pauses or arrest. A sinus exit block happens if the T cells can't send the signal to the rest of the heart.

The treatment is to determine if there is a reversible cause of this problem (like drugs or electrolyte disturbances) and fix it. A pacemaker might be necessary. Most people with sinus node dysfunction do well, even if they aren't treated with a pacemaker. The risk of sudden cardiac death from this problem is very low.

Premature Atrial Contractions

Premature atrial contractions or PACs begin in the atria but not in the SA node. There are many reasons for having these, including drugs and medications, structural heart problems, and several medical diseases. Many are idiopathic with no known cause. Some actually come from the area of the pulmonary veins. PACs look a lot like regular P waves and QRS complexes. They come earlier than expected, with a space after that before a regular beat kicks in. The P wave may not look like normal:

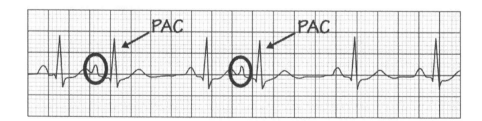

If you see PACs, think of these possibilities:

- *Is there a structural problem with the heart?* This can include anything wrong with the atria, ventricles, or coronary arteries.
- *Are there chemical causes?* These can include medicines for depression, anything that activates the sympathetic nervous system, digoxin, and chemotherapy drugs.
- *Is there a disease causing this?* This might include heart attacks, COPD, diabetes, heart failure, or high blood pressure.

- *Is there something else?* These include pregnancy, anxiety, tobacco or alcohol use, or fatigue. Oddly, caffeine is not a cause of this.

PACs are rarely dangerous, but to those who have them, they will be annoying or anxiety-provoking when they are felt as palpitations in the chest. These extra beats do not have to be treated with anything unless they are too symptomatic.

Stop any causative drug and fix any underlying health condition. Beta-blocking drugs and certain drugs used for other heart rhythm disturbances might work. Rarely, a specialist can find the area causing the heart problem and zap it with electrocautery or other treatments to "ablate" or kill off the offending area.

Wandering atrial pacemaker

A wandering atrial pacemaker or WAP is easy to identify. The person looks like they have a normal sinus rhythm until you look at the P waves. They will not look the same over time or even from beat to beat. This is because the source of the beat in the atrium is not the same. It "wanders," exactly as it sounds.

Look for P waves (more noticeable in lead II) that are differently shaped over time. It will be seen in athletes, young people, or the elderly. Most people don't know they have it.

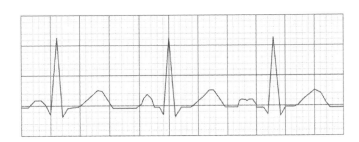

See how funky these P waves are? They are not the same from beat to beat, and the PR intervals will also not be the same.

Atrial fibrillation

Atrial fibrillation is prevalent—and very dangerous to the walking, talking person who has it. The atria have given up having a P wave at all, so you'll only see a fibrillating, wavy background on the isoelectric line. If you looked at the heart, you wouldn't see beating atria. They would quiver instead. There are multiple tiny areas of electrical activity in the atrium, all contributing in some small way to the atria's output. It might look like this:

A Fib

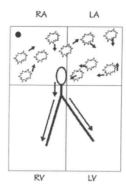

Most people who have it will have a too fast heart rate, some with short episodes while others have it persistently. The reason it is dangerous is that blood pools in the atria and clots there. When these clots eventually break off, some may go to the brain, leading to a stroke. The highest risk person is one who has atrial fibrillation long enough for clotting to occur before they flip back into normal sinus rhythm. This jarring change causes the clots to break off easily.

Who gets atrial fibrillation or AFib? Usually, those who have structural heart problems, high blood pressure, lung disease, a history of alcohol use, or are very elderly. If there are symptoms, it usually comes from the rapid heartbeat, leading to chest pain, fainting, shortness of breath, palpitations, sweating, nausea, or dizziness. This is what AFib looks like:

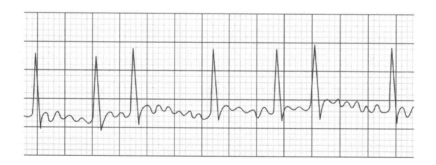

Atrial fibrillation generally needs to be treated. This is done in several ways:

- You can slow the heart rate down to acceptable levels.
- You can shock the heart or "cardiovert" it to a normal rhythm.
- You can give anticoagulant drugs to prevent blood clots.
- You can kill off or ablate the part of the heart causing the problem.
- You can put in a pacemaker that overrides the rapid atrial rate.

One thing for sure: even if the person with atrial fibrillation seems normal or unaffected, he or she has a higher risk for stroke, and this risk must be managed.

Atrial flutter

This is almost as common as atrial fibrillation. The individual with atrial flutter will have an ECG with a characteristic "saw-tooth" pattern. The atrial rate will be very fast, up to 300 bpm. The good news is that these do not get transmitted on a beat-to-beat basis. If it did, your heart would fail quickly, because the ventricles wouldn't have a chance to fill with each beat. This would just be messy and not compatible with life at all.

In atrial flutter, there is a circular electrical activity pattern in the atria that causes repeated impulses to be sent down to the AV node. It looks a great deal like this:

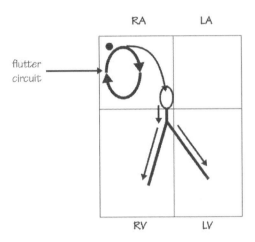

A Flutter

The ventricular rate will generally be half, a third or a fourth of the atrial rate, because every second through fourth beat or so is picked up as the AV node gets out of its refractory period and accepts/transmits one of the atrial beats.

This kind of rhythm is called a reentry arrhythmia because the same pattern gets "recycled" beat after beat, with no chance for the normal rhythm to establish itself.

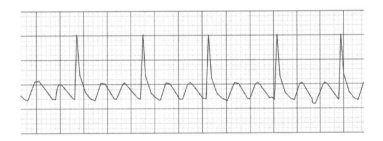

The rhythm shown is atrial fibrillation with 3:1 conduction, because the ventricles capture every third atrial beat. You have to assume that there is a P wave hidden beneath the QRS complex. Depending on the person's symptoms and other factors, you would treat this by controlling the rate, giving blood thinners, or converting the rhythm to normal sinus rhythm with cardioversion.

Paroxysmal atrial tachycardia

As you'll soon see, there are a lot of atrial-type rhythms that can all be called "supraventricular tachycardia." These can be confusing because they are so similar. Atrial tachycardia is a type of SVT that doesn't have any accessory pathways in the heart. The QRS will be narrow with a heart rate between 100 and 250 bpm. The shape of the P wave varies. It can be seen in people with normal and abnormal heart structures.

Look for some noncardiac cause of the problem, such as a release of adrenaline, low blood oxygen levels, alcohol or drug use, electrolyte imbalance, and exercise. As a type of SVT, atrial tachycardia isn't very common. The source of the P wave does not have to be the SA node. As you can see, it is called "paroxysmal" because it just jumps in there and then jumps back out:

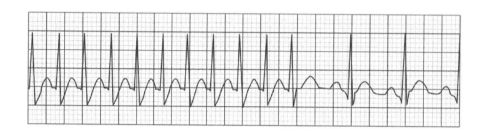

You would treat paroxysmal atrial tachycardia if it was long-lasting and had a rapid rate. Adenosine IV will often stop this rhythm cold, but you might need to consider cardioversion if this doesn't work. There are other choices, too, like beta-blockers, diltiazem, or verapamil that might help.

Multifocal atrial tachycardia

This is called MAT and is another type of supraventricular tachycardia. The main feature is that there are multiple foci in the atria where the P waves originate. The heart rate will be fast, and the P waves will be different. At least three different P waves not from the SA node must be seen in the same lead to make the diagnosis. The PR intervals and PP intervals will be different across the reading.

MAT is seen with older people who have COPD. It can also be seen in those with low potassium and magnesium levels. It is mostly asymptomatic and doesn't need treatment. The biggest risk is with people who have this as part of an acute illness. It still doesn't need treatment but indicates an increase in death in the affected person. Look for it in severe lung disease or in cases where a respiratory arrest is imminent.

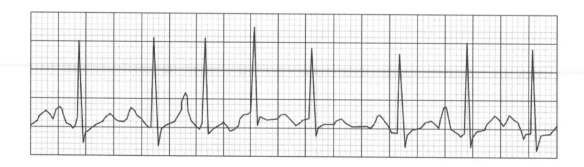

See how different the P waves are in this example? This leads to differences in the R-R interval and an irregular heart rate.

Most of these cases get better on their own. The goal of treatment is to see if there is any reversible condition causing this, such as low electrolyte levels. Magnesium is especially good at correcting these types of rhythm disturbances. Beta-blocker drugs will help reduce the excessive sympathetic nervous system stimulation these people often have. In rare cases, you can do ablation of the hyperactive areas. The downside of this is that you will cause heart block that needs to be managed with a pacemaker.

Did you know? *While MAT is usually a benign heart finding, if you go to the hospital with any type of acute illness and your doctor finds a new onset of MAT, you only have a 40 percent chance of ever getting out of the hospital alive. If you do pull through, the average lifespan after that is just a year.*

Paroxysmal supraventricular tachycardia

Paroxysmal supraventricular tachycardia or PSVT is another type of SVT. It comes on suddenly and usually resolves by itself. The heart rate is regular in this type of rhythm. You will see this in all ages, and you will find it hard to treat. This is because it tends to come on suddenly and is usually so brief. The discussion is really about prevention rather than treatment.

PSVT has many causes, including caffeine, elevated thyroid conditions, nicotine, and several heart-related drugs. Illicit drugs can cause this, including cocaine, amphetamines, and ecstasy. Too much alcohol can lead to PSVT. Serious heart and lung diseases can affect the heart, so that PSVT is more common. Being dehydrated, low in oxygen, or anxious can lead to this rhythm problem.

PSVT is a reentry arrhythmia. This is basically a circle that goes back to the atria, restimulating the areas of the heart through a pathway that overrides the normal sinus node to the AV node pathway. It looks a great deal like this:

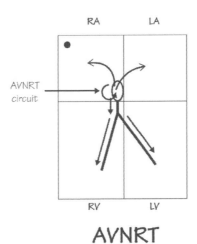

AVNRT

The ECG tracing will be very characteristic and will show this rapid regular rhythm. It often looks like this:

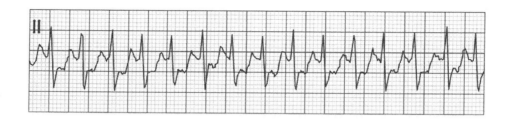

If you feel thoroughly confused about these rapid rhythm disorders, fear not. Most of the distinctions between things like PSVT, PAT, and AVNRT (AV nodal reentrant tachycardia) are meaningless. They look the same on an ECG. It is more important to distinguish things like atrial flutter and PSVT, for example. Here is a brief summary:

Name of Disorder	Heart Rate	P Waves
Sinus tachycardia	Greater than 100 bpm	Normal
Atrial tachycardia	120-150 bpm	Not from SA node
MAT	120-200 bpm	Greater than 3 different P waves
Atrial flutter	200-300 bpm	Sawtooth pattern
Atrial fibrillation	Variable	None visible
AVNRT/PSVT/PAT	150-250 bpm	Short PR interval

WPW syndrome

WPW or Wolff-Parkinson-White is a congenital disease that comes from a known abnormal accessory pathway in the heart. It can be very life-threatening. The PR interval is short and the QRS is long, with a delta wave or slurred upstroke at the beginning of the QRS complex. The rate will be fast, so the patient may feel dizzy, light-headed, or like they might faint.

The impulse to the ventricles comes from the atria but bypasses the AV node entirely. The impulse you see is a fusion of the normal and accessory pathways. The person has both a reentrant tachycardia and a pre-excitation tachycardia. The pre-excitation part is where the delta wave comes from. It is complicated. You need to understand that both of these pathways exist:

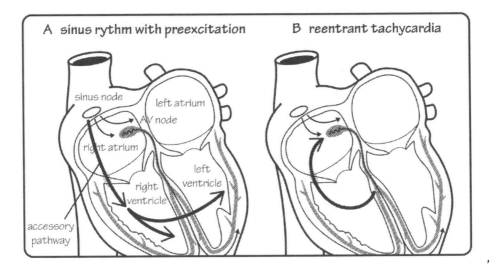

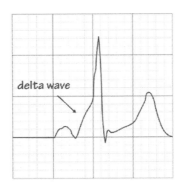

Your ECG will be characteristic and look like this:

Not everyone with WPW will know they have it, because they have never experienced a rapid heart rate. If there are never any symptoms, the disease doesn't have to be treated. If there are tachyarrhythmias, there is preventative medication to take.

Junctional Rhythms

When we talk about "junctional" anything in ECG terms, we mean the AV node. It is the junction between the atria and ventricles and is where the electrical signal takes a little break, so that the ventricles can fill before contracting again. When it comes to the ECG, this is where the QRS complex begins to widen, differentiating an atrial and ventricular source of the heartbeat.

If a rhythm is junctional, the origin is in the AV node itself, or the upper part of the bundle of His. There are several junctional rhythms you might encounter. What you call it depends almost exclusively on the heart rate you see. These are your choices:

- Junctional bradycardia—less than 40 bpm
- Junctional escape rhythm—40-60 bpm
- Accelerated junctional rhythm—60-100 bpm
- Junctional tachycardia—greater than 100 bpm

These rhythms happen when the AV node has more automaticity than the SA node, or when the SA node is blocked in some way. There are numerous reasons for this problem. Sick sinus syndrome could cause it; many medications for the heart are potentially causative. Inflammatory diseases like Lyme disease and rheumatic fever need to be considered. Heart attacks, anorexia nervosa, sleep apnea, and hypoxia are potential causes. The most common cause is sick sinus syndrome, seen in 1 out of 600 older individuals. Athletes with high vagal tone can show this while sleeping.

The QRS will be fairly narrow if the AV node is the source of this rhythm. You won't see any P waves, or you will see upside-down P waves, which happen because of the retrograde flow of electricity up from the AV node to the SA node. This is a strip without any P waves:

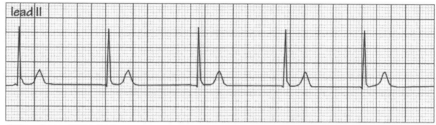

You have to be careful when treating this rhythm. You don't want to affect the AV node's electricity because this is a necessary escape rhythm. Without its activity, you will only have asystole or an even slower rate originating further down the heart's electrical pathway. Do not treat anyone without symptoms. Remove causative medications and treat any underlying causes of this problem but don't mess with the heart itself if you don't have to.

Junctional tachycardia

Junctional tachycardia is also called JET, which stands for junctional ectopic tachycardia. It is seen more often in babies or kids. The AV node is the origin of the beat. Most of the time, it is congenital and might even be seen at the time of birth. In cases of heart defects repaired after birth, it can be seen exclusively in the postoperative setting. Both of these conditions are quite rare.

The main problem here is that the AV node is too "automatic," so it has greater automaticity than the SA node. This is why the rate is so fast and why drugs normally used to stop this type of rhythm do not work. There are no drugs that can block this differential between the AV nodal automaticity and the SA nodal automaticity. This is a genetic problem that essentially can't be fixed.

This is what JET looks like:

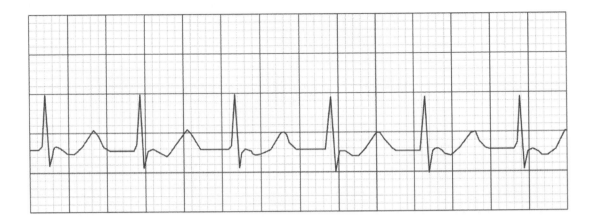

Note the lack of P waves and the rapid rate, which together define this problem.

The problem isn't entirely benign. Babies can have heart rates in the 200-250 bpm minute range, even before birth. The baby who has this can have heart failure and can die in utero, because the heart rate is simply too fast. After birth, babies will have a risk for ventricular fibrillation or complete heart block, leading to sudden death from these arrhythmias. Years ago, about a third of all babies died from this problem; nowadays it is fewer than 10 percent.

To treat this problem, babies can receive drugs like amiodarone to block it, or other antiarrhythmic drugs can be used. Look for problems with electrolytes being too high or too low, and fix it if you see it. No matter how you treat this issue, it is very hard to correct unless it happens after surgery. Postoperative JET usually gets better by itself.

Premature junctional contractions

Premature junctional contractions or PJCs are really nothing special, simply extra beats coming from the AV node or just beneath it. They can be seen in a healthy person and in sick people who have some problem with their heart (like valvular disease or toxicity from medications). Immersion in cold water will also cause PJCs. It is called a junctional rhythm if there are more than two beats in a row. The QRS will be fairly narrow but will not have a P wave causing it.

Premature Ventricular Contractions

These are called PVCs or ventricular premature beats (VPBs). They are very common and not always pathological. If they are frequent and occur with known heart disease, the frequency predicts disease progression and a worsened outcome. These can also cause heart failure if too frequent.

PVCs look different, depending on where they come from in the heart. Because they are beyond the AV node, the QRS will almost always be wide. The 12-lead ECG can help you identify where the ventricular beat is coming from. Left ventricular beats will naturally show a blockage of the right bundle branch and vice versa.

Where do these come from? Some are due to excessive stimulation of the sympathetic nervous system. Illicit drug use of things like cocaine, amphetamines, or alcohol can contribute to PVCs. Many medications will cause these too, like tricyclic antidepressants, caffeine, and aminophylline. Low blood oxygen or high blood carbon dioxide (CO_2) levels cause frequent PVCs. Any type of heart disease, including heart attacks or inflammation of the heart, make the heart more irritable, leading to PVCs. They can be seen in the normal population (less than 2 percent of the time) but are much more frequent in those who have known heart disease.

PVCs come from a site in the ventricles with increased irritability and automaticity. Electrolyte imbalances, myocardial ischemia, and high adrenergic states will all cause increased automaticity. Reentry circumstances can also cause PVCs in some circumstances. When you do an ECG, expect them to look like this:

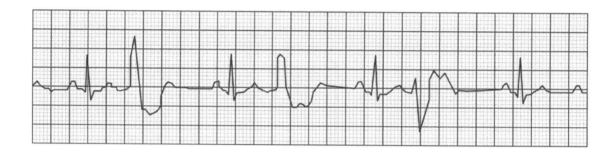

This image is a bit of a trick; this is not just frequent PVCs but is called ventricular bigeminy. Bigeminy is when every other beat is a PVC, while ventricular trigeminy is a PVC every third beat. You do not need to treat them unless they are symptomatic or have runs of PVCs in a row. The risk of runs of these beats is ventricular tachycardia and ventricular fibrillation, both of which are very dangerous.

Ventricular tachycardia

VTach or ventricular tachycardia involves groupings of PVCs in a row, with each beat having a QRS complex of more than 120 ms, and a rate greater than 100 bpm. Sustained VTach lasts longer than 30 seconds, while non-sustained VTach lasts less. The longer it lasts, the greater the risk of hemodynamic instability/shock.

You can also define VTach in other ways. If all of the QRS complexes are the same, it is called monomorphic VTach:

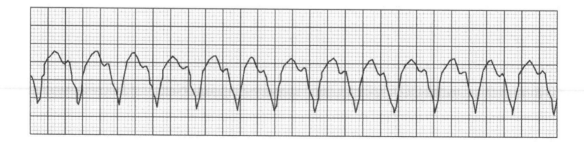

If the QRS complexes are different, it is called polymorphic VTach. There is a type of VTach called Torsades de Pointes, which is polymorphic. In Torsades de Pointes, the QT interval will be long.

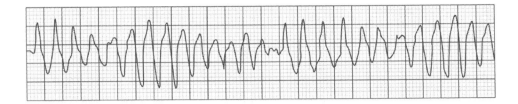

Did you know? *Torsades de Pointes has a funny name because it was discovered by a French physician named François Dessertenne in 1966. He called this Torsades de Pointes or "twisting of the peaks" because of the appearance of twisted QRS complexes.*

There is another type called bidirectional VTach, seen with an alternation of QRS complexes from beat to beat, in cases of drug toxicity from digitalis. Most people with VTach have ischemic heart disease. It is one of the more common rhythms seen in a person who has collapsed from cardiac arrest.

The treatment depends on whether or not the person is stable. Unstable VTach is treated just like VFib—just shock/defibrillate until you get a better, more perfusable rhythm. A person stable enough to have a pulse and blood pressure is treated with drugs to convert their rhythm to something more normal. Procainamide is the drug of choice because it works up to 80 percent of the time. Amiodarone works about 30 percent of the time. You can also use cardioversion. People who frequently develop this rhythm often need an implantable cardioverter/defibrillator device.

Did you know? *What is the difference between cardioversion and defibrillation? Defibrillation is mainly done with VFib, basically a random shocking of the heart. Cardioversion is gentler and involves a lesser amount of applied electricity for each shock. The shock is timed carefully to be given without the potential for creating a worsened rhythm by applying the shock at the wrong time.*

Idioventricular rhythm

Idioventricular rhythm is basically VTach in slow motion. The heart rate is less than 50 bpm, the QRS interval is long, and you'll find no P waves. These are actually the escape rhythm patterns of the ventricles. It can be called accelerated when the heart rate is 50-110 bpm. Most of the time, these are stable rhythms from a hemodynamic standpoint. The person will be walking with a perfusable blood pressure. Here is an example of accelerated idioventricular rhythm:

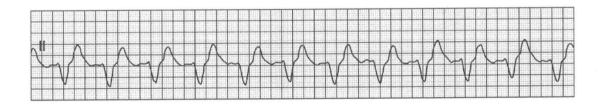

In most cases of accelerated idioventricular rhythm, the person has a high parasympathetic tone to their heart and a low sympathetic tone. Look for it when the AV node is completely blocked, and when the AV node itself can't make a normal escape rhythm. You will see it after the heart is reperfused following a heart attack, when certain drugs are taken in excess, in babies with heart defects, or in athletes.

Most people don't need treatment, as it will resolve when you remove the underlying cause. If the heart rate is too slow or fast, there are drugs to control it. Amiodarone or lidocaine might help the rhythm problem itself. If the rate is too slow, consider a pacemaker.

Ventricular fibrillation

Ventricular fibrillation is the most common rhythm disturbance you'll see in a witnessed cardiac arrest. It usually is when the rhythm has started as VTach but then degenerated into a coarser and coarser picture that doesn't resemble much after true VFib has been discovered. It is rare in children but more common among people with heart disease. Most who have this will have coronary artery disease and a heart attack.

Ventricular fibrillation is also characteristic and is seen as a squiggly line with no P waves or QRS complexes. It can be arbitrarily determined to be "coarse" or "fine." There are multiple reentrant pathways and repolarizations happening throughout the ventricular myocardium. Your main recourse to establish a normal rhythm is to defibrillate.

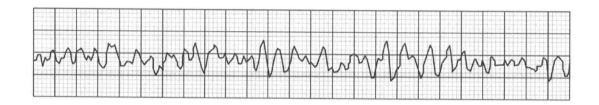

This is coarse VFib, which will gradually degenerate further into fine VTach and then asystole.

Asystole

Asystole is bad; there are no two ways around it. The only time asystole isn't bad is when your ECG malfunctioning causes it. If you see asystole on a rhythm strip, check another lead or a 12-lead ECG to confirm this isn't the problem. If you see it in all leads, the person is largely dead, with a survival rate of about 10 percent at a hospital and 0-2 percent outside one. Kids and hypothermic patients have the best overall chance of making it.

It is easy to identify once you have determined it is real. It's basically a flat line:

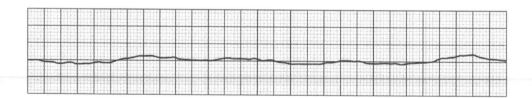

Resuscitation outside of a hospital is very difficult. You can try to shock them, but there often isn't enough electrical energy within the heart to draw from to get a perfusable rhythm. However, there are some underlying correctible causes that might help, provided you can correct them quickly enough. The people who wrote the ACLS (Advanced Cardiac Life Support) protocol have several ideas for why systole might be present. These are called the Hs and Ts:

Hs in Asystole	Ts in Asystole
Hypoxia	Tension pneumothorax
Acidosis (low hydrogen)	Cardiac tamponade
Hypokalemia	Toxins
Hyperkalemia	Pulmonary thrombosis
Hypothermia	Coronary thrombosis

Even among those with inpatient cardiac arrests, the rate of survival is low. Cold patients with hypothermia do better than warm patients. The cause is mostly due to extra-cardiac reasons, leading to a failure of any intrinsic electrical activity to be generated in the heart. The muscle is not perfused much, so the patient largely dies of this in short order.

The treatment is to start CPR while looking for reversible causes. Get arterial blood gases and a potassium level STAT. Vasopressin and epinephrine have been used, but their effectiveness is questionable. Many doctors use transcutaneous pacing techniques, which rarely help improve survival. If efforts are tried and fail, this would be a good time to stop, call the cardiac arrest, and declare the patient dead.

To Sum Things Up

There are many different cardiac arrhythmias, and they do not have to be too confusing once you determine where in the heart it is coming from. The main sources of arrhythmias are the atria, the AV node, and the ventricles. Keep these in mind when you analyze a 12-lead ECG or rhythm strip. Once you identify the disturbance, think of the potential causes of the arrhythmia, and seek out a solution first—even before correcting the disturbance urgently, unless the disturbance is dangerous by itself.

So far, we have talked about the major disturbances you'll see. The ones we haven't talked about yet are the conduction blocks, which are rhythm changes seen when there is a major blockage in the heart. Some are found incidentally, while others are more ominous and symptomatic.

CHAPTER 5:
CONDUCTION BLOCKS

We talked earlier about conduction blocks, but this chapter will go into them in greater detail, so you can recognize them clearly on an ECG and understand why it looks the way it does. When it comes to these types of blocks, it's important to remember that it can be anywhere from the SA node to the Purkinje fibers.

While you'll see that most conduction blocks come from an ischemic event such as a myocardial infarction, which disrupts the pathway if it is strategically placed in one of the heart's major electrical pathways, this is not universally true. There can be other types of disruptions that block the pathways but do not involve ischemia or infarction of heart conduction cells.

Atrioventricular (AV) blocks

These types of blocks are self-explanatory, even though there is more than one type of AV block. The pathway disrupted is between the SA node (the atrium) and the AV node (ventricular gateway). Because this area is represented by the space between the P wave and the QRS complex, this is exactly where you need to look for the abnormality.

You should expect to see a normal P wave and QRS complex in every lead. Every P wave should a QRS that follows it, and the PR interval should be normal (120 – 200 ms) and the same for every heartbeat. If you don't see that, it's correct to suspect some type of AV conduction block.

AV blocks may be temporary or permanent. They can be due to some anatomic blockage or a "functional blockage," in which there might be an electrolyte disturbance leading to a transient blockage of this normal pathway.

There are four types of AV blocks you should be able to identify easily. Some are from high degrees of vagal tone affecting the heart, and show areas of fibrosis or scar tissue in the conduction system. About 40 percent are due to ischemia of the heart in the affected area. Young people with hypertrophy of the heart due to hypertrophic myopathy might also have an AV block. Infiltrative diseases like amyloidosis and sarcoidosis involve protein deposits in the heart and elsewhere that can damage the AV nodal pathways. And some infections and autoimmune diseases will affect the heart as well.

As you can see from this image, there is no "straight shot" from the SA node to the AV node. The SA node spreads its electrical message far and wide, with some of this message reaching the AV node:

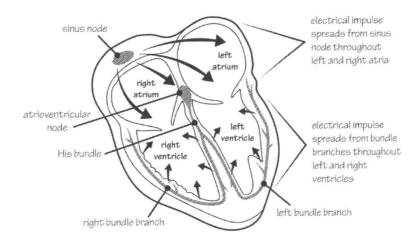

The four different AV node conduction delays occur in different parts of the pathway from the SA node downward. Depending on what you see, you can expect the blockage to be in one of four different areas:

- First-degree AV block—AV node or left atrium
- Second-degree AV block (type I)—AV node
- Second-degree AV block (type II)—bundle His below the AV node
- Third-degree AV block—anywhere at or below the AV node

First-degree AV block

A first-degree AV block is easy to spot. There will be P waves and QRS complexes with no skipped or dropped beats. The only way to recognize it is to measure the PR interval. If it is longer than 200 ms, this is a first-degree AV block. This is due to a minor blockage between the SA node and the AV node. If the PR interval is too long, the P wave will be hidden in the previous T wave and will be hard to see. It looks like this:

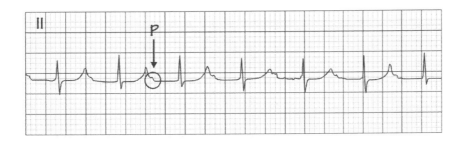

Some people have first-degree AV block as a normal part of their ECG. An inferior MI or increased vagal tone among athletes can both cause first-degree AV block. Certain drugs and high potassium levels can also cause this. In almost all situations, this type of AV block is not treated and has no symptoms.

Second-degree AV block

A second-degree AV block, regardless of type, is considered an incomplete AV block. The connection between the SA node and AV node is sometimes present, but not always.

You might see one out of every few P waves picked up to make a QRS complex. You can also see a more complex pattern, such is seen in Mobitz type I disease.

Type I or Mobitz I Disease

Mobitz I or Wenckebach AV block is a more benign type of second-degree AV block. The PR interval is not the same for each beat. The best way to identify this is by using calipers. Find a short-appearing PR interval and set its length with the calipers. Then check the PR intervals of the next few beats. If these are getting progressively longer, suspect type I AV blockage.

At some point, the calipers will run across a P wave for which there is no QRS seen. This dropped event signifies that this is definitely Wenckebach. You will also notice that the PR interval after the dropped QRS complex is narrow again. You cannot predict how long this run of prolonged PR intervals will be before one P wave isn't conducted.

This is better appreciated on a longer rhythm strip where you can see the pattern more clearly. The PP intervals will be the same throughout, and the greatest change in PR intervals is seen at the beginning of the cycle, becoming less noticeable over time.

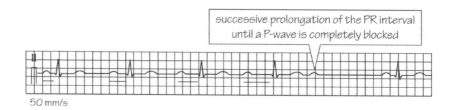

successive prolongation of the PR interval until a P-wave is completely blocked

50 mm/s

Most of the time, this is reversible and occurs at the level of the AV node. There is no damage to the AV nodal cells; they just become increasingly tired of passing on the P wave until one is dropped. This is partly why it is considered relatively benign, even though it can be seen in an injured heart with reversible ischemia or inflammation. The increased vagal tone of athletes will also cause this pattern, and some heart medications will contribute to seeing this as well.

People with Mobitz I arrhythmia will rarely have symptoms, and will not often progress to higher AV nodal blockade degrees. For this reason, it does not often require treatment. Because it is a reversible phenomenon, you can remove the cause (such as an offending medication), and the disturbance will disappear.

Type II or Mobitz II Disease

You can identify Mobitz type II disease because both the PR interval and the PP interval are the same throughout. The RR intervals will not be the same because, every so often, the QRS complex is dropped. The distance between the QRS complexes on either side of the dropped beat will be precisely twice the RR interval of the normal beats. This type of AV block is also called a Hay block.

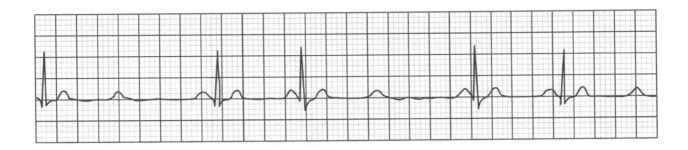

This blockage is further down the conduction pathway than Mobitz I, often below the AV node itself. The conduction cells don't tire out; they simply suddenly refuse to pass along the impulse. The problem is rarely functional or physiological, but rather usually due to structural disease of the affected area. The problem can also be due to prior infarction or fibrosis/scar tissue in the conduction system.

The QRS complex can be wide and strange-appearing because the defect is below the AV node. There might be a pattern when the dropped QRS complex is seen, but this doesn't have to be the case. An anterior MI can cause this, but so can heart inflammation or fibrosis due to any cause. High potassium can contribute to this, and some drugs will be causative.

Depending on how many beats are dropped, the bradycardia and symptoms can be severe. There is a high likelihood of progression to complete heart block compared to Mobitz I disease. Asystole can come from this rhythm, which would almost certainly be fatal. This needs to be managed with a pacemaker to avoid a fatal complication. Medications like atropine used for Mobitz I disease will make people with Mobitz II disease worse.

Did you know? *Atropine is one of the few drugs that will increase the heart rate. It does this by blocking the muscarinic/parasympathetic receptors in the SA node. This dials down the heart's parasympathetic influence, leaving behind more of a sympathetic influence, which raises the heart rate by increasing the firing rate of the SA node.*

There is a type of second-degree AV block that looks and acts much like a third-degree block, because more than one P wave in a row will be blocked. It's easy to see how dangerous this is, because it means it is harder to get the impulse down the entire conduction pathway. The blockage is below the AV node, and the ventricular rate is slow enough to be very symptomatic. You will still see a relationship between some P waves and some QRS complexes.

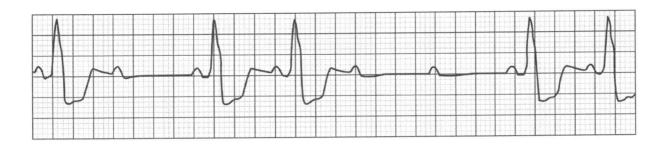

Third-degree AV block

This is also called complete heart block. There is no transmission of the P wave through the AV node, so there will be regular P waves and regular QRS complexes but no relationship between the two waveforms. The ventricular conduction happens only because of some type of slow junctional or ventricular escape rhythms. As you know, escape rhythms tend to be very slow and are the heart's last-ditch effort to get a rhythm going.

Complete heart block usually comes from the worsening of a Mobitz II second-degree block. If you see a junctional escape rhythm, the damage is above the AV node. If the QRS complexes are wider and slower, the damage is below the AV node. The rate can be as slow as 20-40 bpm if the escape rhythm comes from the ventricles (below the AV node).

Of course, the risk is that this will go on to asystole without warning. An MI can cause this (especially an inferior one), as well as drugs, as can anything that degenerates the conducting system cells.

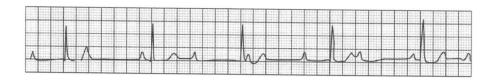

One strange thing you might see is called complete AV dissociation. This is also related to a dissociation between the atria and ventricles, but the ventricular rate is actually faster than the SA nodal rate. This is due to the irritability of the ventricles, which will beat faster than the atria.

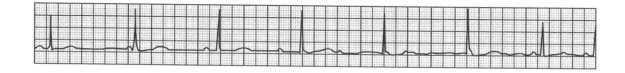

If an AV nodal blockage needs treatment at all, the main treatment used will be pacing. Pacing the heart can be temporary or permanent. Atropine can be used in some cases, but it doesn't last long and will worsen the situation for many of these patients.

Bundle branch blocks

Remember that the electrical conducting system goes down the septum as the bundle of His, which goes quickly into a left and right bundle branch. The left bundle branch goes to the left ventricle, while the right goes to the right. Blockages of the bundle branches are harder to spot than the AV blocks, but there are some clues you can use.

Right Bundle Branch Block (RBBB)

This involves a blockage of the right His-Purkinje system of the heart. The QRS will be wide, and you'll recognize it according to which leads are most affected. The major coronary artery (left anterior descending) supplies this area, along with one circumflex branch. There are two circumflex branches available (right and left), but which one supplies this area depends on the person and which vessel is dominant in their heart.

An RBBB can be caused by any type of ischemia, including those caused by having a right heart catheterization, which will affect the blood supply to this part of the heart. If you see this in the setting of a heart attack, expect a greater chance of death, but if seen as an isolated event it is not considered dangerous.

Here's how you identify an RBBB:

1. Look for a QRS complex longer than 120 ms (remember that the left ventricle depolarizes first and then the right). When there is a delay of one ventricle, the QRS complex will be wider.
2. Look in the precordial leads V1 and V2 for an RSR' wave.

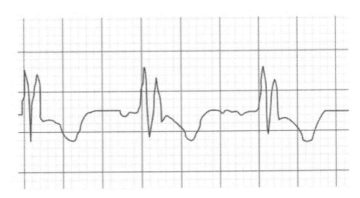

3. Look in all precordial leads for a longer S wave than the R wave *or* for an S wave longer than 40 ms.

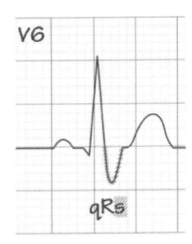

4. Look for an R wave peak time of longer than 50 ms in lead V1, but normal peak times for the R wave in the lateral leads (V5 and V6).
5. Look for inverted T waves on the right precordial leads, but upright T waves in the left precordial leads.

An RBBB by itself does not have to be treated unless the ejection fraction is low in heart failure. Then you would do resynchronization of the heart.

Left Bundle Branch Block

A left bundle branch block or LBBB is more common than an RBBB. Most people who have this have a great deal of heart disease, but this isn't universally true. If it is isolated without heart disease, it is nothing to be concerned about. However, if it is seen in the setting of chest pain thought to be heart-related, it can by itself indicate that an MI has occurred.

Other causes of an LBBB include dilation of the heart, as you'll see in cardiomyopathy. This stretches the fibers of the conducting system and may damage them. Remember that many things will enlarge the heart, including inflammation, infarction, valvular disease, and infections of the heart. When in doubt, however, suspect infarction first.

The left bundle branch block can be determined on an ECG using these criteria:

1. Look for a QRS duration longer than 120 ms.
2. Look for a small R wave and a big S wave *or* a QS wave in V1.

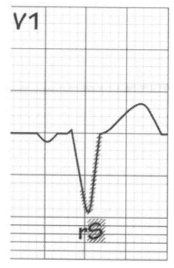

3. Look for a notched R wave and no Q wave in V6.

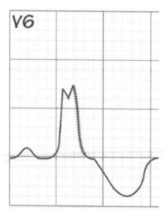

The finding of LBBB does not need to be treated as an isolated event. This is almost always permanent. As with an RBBB, cardiac resynchronization is used if the person has heart failure. This is done using a pacemaker that stimulates the right and left ventricles at the same time.

Hemiblocks

Hemiblocks are a very picky definition in the world of ECGs. They involve damage to one of the two fascicles that the left bundle branch breaks into as it descends the interventricular septum. In the heart, these look like this:

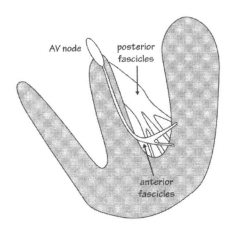

The two fascicles go to different parts of the left ventricle, so they have different meanings when either of them is affected by a blockage. Let's see if these hemiblocks have any real significance.

Left Anterior Fascicular Block

The left anterior fascicular block, also known as the left anterior hemiblock (LAFB/LAHB), can be seen by looking at a couple of things on the 12-lead ECG. First, look at the axis. You should see a left axis deviation of more than -45 degrees.

1. Look on lead III to see if there is a qR complex in lead I and an rS complex in lead III.
2. Look on leads II, III and aVF (inferior leads) for an rS complex.

An LAFB/LAHB occurs when the anterior fascicle of the left bundle branch is no longer able to conduct action potentials. The criteria to diagnose a LAFB or LAHB on an ECG include:

1. Left axis deviation of at least -45 degrees
2. The presence of a qR complex in lead I (notice the tiny q wave and the bigger R wave)

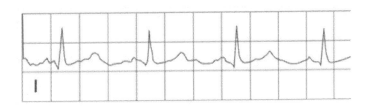

3. Usually an rS complex in lead II and III (sometimes aVF as well [notice the large S wave and the tiny r wave])

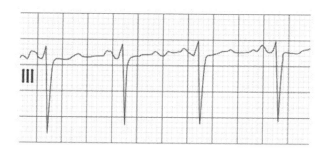

Anytime you see a large left axis deviation, look for an upright QRS complex in lead I and a downward QRS complex in lead aVF. Then notice the rS complex in lead III as shown. This will quickly lead you to the correct diagnosis.

If you see these findings, it's important to note that if the patient has an old inferior MI, you will not be able to tell this easily. This is because there will be Q waves inferiorly already because of the hemiblock, masking any Q waves due to an old myocardial infarction.

Left Posterior Fascicular Block

This is abbreviated as LPHB or LPFB. It isn't as commonly seen as a LAFB would be. It involves damage or blockage in the left posterior fascicle of the left ventricle. It isn't as common because the fibers of this fascicle are spread out; it means you'd have to have a big heart attack or other illness to damage this expanded area of the heart. Other criteria when looking for an LPFB include:

1. The axis will be deviated to the right between 90 and 180 degrees.
2. You will see a qR complex in lead III (notice the small q wave and bigger R wave in this lead).

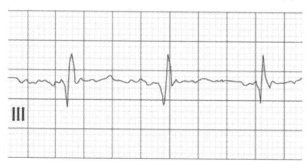

3. You will see an rS in lead I (notice the smaller R wave and bigger S wave in this lead).

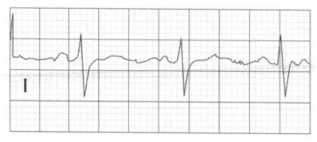

There are even messier situations than this, such as trifascicular blocks and bifascicular blocks. These are important to cardiologists, but don't make much difference to the average ECG technician or ER doctor.

To Sum Things Up

Conduction issues in the heart essentially mean that some type of damage (permanent or temporary) occurred in the conducting cells. Many come from a myocardial infarction, where the cells that would normally conduct the electrical impulses in the heart are dead. This means that the normal pathway for electricity in the heart will not function.

What you'll see on the ECG depends largely on where the blockage is located. AV blocks are relatively common and occur between the SA node and the vicinity of the AV node. Other blockages lower than that will have their own characteristics and significance. The block itself may or may not be significant. If any of these result in bradycardia, the person may not be stable and will faint. Others have few symptoms, but this means something has happened in the affected area that is worrisome.

As always, it is a good idea to look at your patient as a whole being and not just the ECG. It tells you a lot, but if the patient has chest pain, low blood pressure or other symptoms, these are just as important as what you see on the rhythm strip.

CHAPTER 6:
CARDIAC HYPERTROPHY AND ENLARGEMENT

The terms "cardiac hypertrophy" and "cardiac enlargement" can be confusing, and you might be tempted to think they are the same thing when they really aren't. The word "hypertrophy" as applied to the heart means "muscle thickening." You need to see more muscle in the heart to be able to use this term. The ventricles are almost always the source of thickening. There just isn't enough muscle in atrial walls to have the thickening mean much.

Cardiac enlargement, on the other hand, means the heart is bigger. The atria can easily enlarge, especially in atrial fibrillation, when the atria just fill with blood and never contract. The ventricles, too, can simply enlarge without being hypertrophic (thickened). On an x-ray, you will only see a big heart silhouette on the film, showing heart enlargement but not indicating if the muscle is thick or not. You'll need an ECG or other imaging system to tell the difference.

Types of Hypertrophy and Enlargement of the Heart

Diseases of the heart muscle that cause hypertrophy or enlargement of the heart are called cardiomyopathies. Not all cardiomyopathies are the same, and the causes are many. You can have cardiomyopathy from valvular disease, coronary artery disease, and hereditary or congenital disorders. Most of them fit neatly into three main categories: dilated cardiomyopathy, restrictive cardiomyopathy, and hypertrophic cardiomyopathy. Let's look at what to expect from these different subtypes.

These are what these types look like:

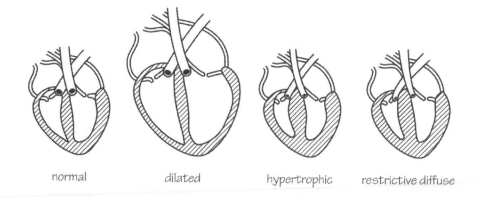

normal   dilated   hypertrophic   restrictive diffuse

Dilated Cardiomyopathy

Dilated cardiomyopathy is probably the most common type you'll encounter. It is seen in people with damaged hearts due to heart disease or valvular disease, which can cause any or all heart chambers to enlarge. Most of these people will eventually develop signs and symptoms of heart failure like shortness of breath, edema of the legs, and difficulty lying flat because of fluid in the lungs. It is usually seen in elderly people.

The key features to remember about this type of cardiomyopathy are that the heart is big and boggy, muscle cells of the heart die off (for various reasons), and the heart wall thins. A thin heart wall will not generate a great deal of extra electricity, so unless there is hypertrophy or heart wall thickening as part of this, you won't see much on an ECG. Depending on the situation, the heart muscle might be thin or thick.

Why would the heart muscle thicken? It's like any other muscle you exercise and try to strengthen. When the heart muscle gets stretched out because there is too much blood in it, it will try to get stronger by thickening the muscle. This is when you'll get hypertrophy of the ventricles, and ECG changes will start to appear.

Common ECG changes you'll see include atrial flutter or atrial fibrillation. This is because the atria do not respond well to being excessively dilated or stretched. They cannot contract and will just fibrillate or quiver. You will also see that the heart is more prone to rapid heart rate rhythms (tachyarrhythmias) before going onto atrial fibrillation. It is hard to get someone out of atrial fibrillation if the atria are too stretched out.

In the ventricles, the chances of hypertrophy are greater. The more pressure in the ventricles, the greater the chance of hypertrophy. Keep in mind that the left ventricle's pressure will be much greater than the right. This means that most of the time, the left ventricle will be thicker than the right. Isolated hypertrophy of the right ventricle is very rare.

Besides heart disease, there are many other causes of dilated cardiomyopathy to think of. Viruses can cause infections of the heart muscle, called viral myocarditis, that destroy enough cells to cause myopathy. Most of these are viruses you likely have never heard of, like coxsackievirus B, but there are more well-known ones such as the HIV virus that can cause infections too. If you've lived or worked in South America, you've probably see lots of Chagas disease-causing cardiomyopathy from infection.

Did you know? *Emotional stress can cause death from cardiomyopathy! It's called takotsubo cardiomyopathy and means "octopus trap" in Japanese, because the doctor who invented the term thought the heart looked a lot like these kinds of traps before the person dies. The stress releases lots of adrenaline and dilates the heart suddenly. This is very bad, so the person dies almost immediately.*

We will talk more about ECG changes in cardiomyopathy in a moment. You may see nothing specific, or you may see things like low voltage (small QRS wave heights), inverted T waves where they shouldn't be, and rapid heart rate. Q waves could be seen. (We haven't talked much about Q waves and what they mean yet, but in this context they really don't mean much.) Of course, you'll also see atrial fibrillation.

Restrictive Cardiomyopathy

Restrictive cardiomyopathy is kind of what it sounds like. The heart muscle is restricted or constrained. It means that during diastole or relaxation of the heart, the heart muscle is too stiff to fill properly. This leads to poor output as well as symptoms like shortness of breath and tiredness. These are hard to treat because the heart muscle is so stiff.

What might cause this kind of stiffness? It's sometimes caused by abnormal substances leaching into the heart muscle tissue. Deposition of amyloid proteins among people with amyloidosis is one reason for stiffness from abnormal substances in the heart. Other systemic diseases like Fabry disease and sarcoidosis cause similar problems.

Muscles are meant to be moveable and elastic, including the heart muscle. If there is scar tissue there or abnormal proteins, these muscles don't really work well. If you've ever seen scar tissue on skin, you know that this tissue isn't very stretchy. In some cases, if a bunch of heart muscle tissue dies off, it is replaced with fibrous tissue or scar tissue (as is true everywhere in the body). The heart doesn't stretch well after that. Once scar tissue forms, it doesn't go away.

If the heart doesn't fill well, the parts trying to pump blood are stressed and have to work harder, including the periphery (or venous system) and the lungs. Both of these are repositories for blood intended to go into the atria. If this can't happen, there is a major blood pileup (not unlike the pileup of cars you'll see on the freeway behind a crash site). You'll see pulmonary venous hypertension and peripheral fluid buildup in the body, depending on where the heart is the stiffest.

So if the person exercises, they will feel short of breath from fluid buildup in the lungs. The pressure in the body's venous system is high enough that liquid from blood spills into the tissues and fluid spaces in the body. Ascites is abdominal fluid in the peritoneal space around the gut; fluid will also go to the ankles and feet, largely because of gravity. Obviously, if you stand all day as part of your job and have restrictive cardiomyopathy, you will have a greater chance of swollen ankles.

As with dilated cardiomyopathy, an ECG will not be beneficial in making the diagnosis. Doctors often call them "nonspecific findings," which usually means there won't be any consistent findings from person to person or that you can't make much of what you are seeing. Q waves, changes in the ST segments, and T wave inversion are probable findings. Different types of blocks, including LBBB or AV blocks, might be seen.

As with dilated cardiomyopathy, the prognosis or outcome for the person with restrictive cardiomyopathy is poor. It's hard to repair this type of damage to the heart, so doctors usually treat the patient's symptoms to try and maintain a good quality of life for as long as possible. Because of frequent heart blocks, you can expect many "sudden cardiac deaths" to come out of having this disorder.

Hypertrophic Cardiomyopathy

Hypertrophic cardiomyopathy is interesting and different from the other two types of cardiomyopathy we've talked about. This is something a person either inherits or is born with. It means that some parts of the heart (usually the left ventricle) are too thick. It isn't often symmetric, so it will not be seen as diffuse thickening of the heart muscle. An accurate picture of a heart with this disorder looks like this:

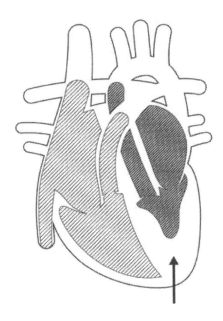

Notice how the right ventricle looks thinner, and how normal it seems compared to the left ventricle, where the muscle is so thick there is barely enough room for the blood to fit.

If you've ever heard of a young teenage athlete dropping dead on the soccer field, you know what happens to some people who have this disorder. A few will have chest pain or shortness of breath, and some will just faint, giving them a chance at surviving this problem. Sadly, those who die suddenly without warning don't have much of a chance.

What kills these young people is a sudden arrhythmia rather than a heart attack. It's why some athletic fields have portable defibrillators handy and why implantable defibrillators are the best cure for people who have this. There are surgeries that can trim off some of the thicker parts of the ventricle that are blocking blood flow out of the heart if it looks like this sort of thing might help.

Because there are more than a thousand variants of this disease, you can expect different ECG findings. This is where you'll really see the ECG effects from a thickened heart muscle. The S wave in V1 added to the R wave in V5 or V6 must be greater than 35 mm. This tracing shows how obvious it can be:

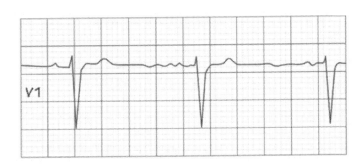
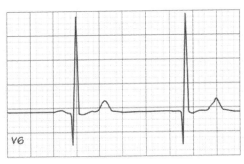

Look also at the Q waves in V6. These "deep Q waves" in the septal leads (I, aVL, V5, and V6) are often seen if the septum between the two ventricles is enlarged. Expect the T waves to be abnormal in some leads as well.

In other cases, the p wave will give the whole thing away. If one atrium is stressed from back pressure in the ventricle, the two p waves won't be the same. Remember, the heart is a lot like a plumbing system. The flow of blood through it must be tightly regulated, because the amount of blood from the left side of the heart must equal blood flow through the right.

If two p waves don't look the same, you'll see a stretched-out or notched p wave—a sure sign the two atria are not doing the same thing at all. The important thing to remember is that you won't likely see this without the other changes seen in the QRS complex. In most cases, the QRS complex will be so abnormally high, it will be obvious on the ECG that hypertrophy is present.

Because this is hereditary, once you've identified a young person with this disorder, you should expect to do ECGs on the siblings of any person identified as having hypertrophic cardiomyopathy or HCM (even though the more appropriate screening test is the echocardiogram). They are most often autosomal dominant in nature, so statistically, half of all siblings could have the disease but might not know it.

Atrial enlargement

Atrial enlargement of the left ventricle comes from excessive filling of this chamber. It was designed to handle a load of blood; however, if a certain limit is reached, the atrium can't contract, and fibrillation occurs as the chamber turns into a big bag of blood that just sits there. It does have some ability to hypertrophy, though, called LAH or left atrial hypertrophy.

As you can imagine, the p wave will be abnormal on the ECG to some degree. Remember that hypertrophy translates into a bigger deflection on the ECG. If you see a bigger p wave "bump" on the first part of the p wave in lead II, it's right atrial hypertrophy, while if it's bigger on the other side it's left. You might see two big bumps if both atria have hypertrophy.

V1 normally has a biphasic p wave so that you can look at the "bump size" on this lead as well. Don't forget that, when you look at an ECG, the left side of the p wave (the first half) represents the right atrium, while the right side of the p wave (the second half) is actually the left side of the patient (and the left atrium). This image explains it all:

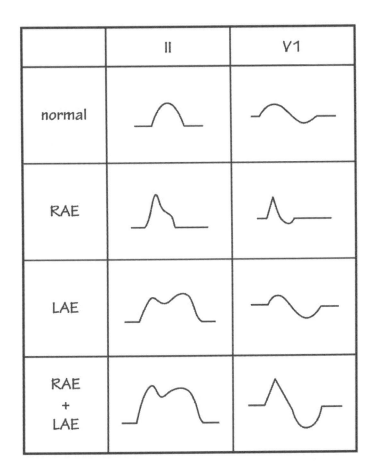

	II	V1
normal		
RAE		
LAE		
RAE + LAE		

The reason you might see LAH by itself is if the person has mitral stenosis. A narrowed mitral valve is rough on the left atrium because it cannot push the blood out fast enough as it contracts, so some doesn't make it into the left ventricle with each beat. Over time, the atrium will hypertrophy to try and overcome the blockage. If this doesn't work, the next step is atrial fibrillation.

On the other hand, left atrial hypertrophy can also be seen along with left ventricular hypertrophy. In severe systemic hypertension, aortic stenosis, hypertrophic cardiomyopathy, or mitral regurgitation, you might see both LVH and LAH together. In this case, the mitral valve is leaky and not blocked, but the effect is the same. In both cases, the pressure inside the left atrium is just too great, so the chamber walls thicken in response to this.

Ventricular Hypertrophy

You probably have a good idea by now what left ventricular hypertrophy (LVH) looks like. The problem is that the ECG by itself isn't a sensitive enough test for LVH, so misses diagnosing half of all cases. However, if you see it on ECG, you can be 90 percent sure or more that it's real.

The basics to look out for are the large QRS amplitude, left axis deviation, and what's called a left ventricular strain pattern. This is a common term with specific criteria you should understand. It usually refers to the ST segment and means that it downslopes into an upside-down T wave. This will be opposite to the main direction of the QRS in the lead you are looking at. It can look like this:

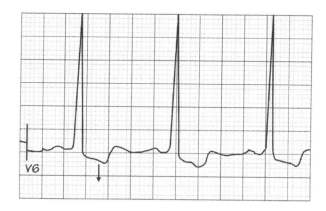

A left ventricular strain pattern is common in LVH, but it can also be seen in ischemic heart disease, which we'll talk about soon.

Several groups have set up established criteria for LVH. There are points given, for example, for having QRS findings, ST-segment changes, evidence of LAH, and left axis deviation on the ECG. Almost all of these criteria show poor sensitivity but good specificity in detecting LVH.

What if it's the right ventricle that is hypertrophied? This isn't as common, but if you see it, you'll see these things:

- Right axis deviation
- Strain pattern in the ST segment
- Tall R waves in the right-handed leads and steep S waves in the lefthanded leads
- Possible incomplete RBBB (a qR seen in lead V1)
- Signs of RAH (as we've talked about)
- Slightly wide QRS complex

For both LVH and RVH, you should look at the precordial leads. If the problem of QRS height is on the patient's right (V1-V3), it will be right ventricular hypertrophy. If the problem is on the patient's left (leads V4-V6), it will be left ventricular hypertrophy. This ECG, for example, shows RVH:

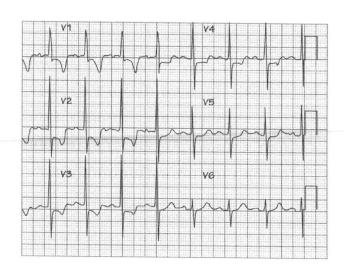

To Sum Things Up

As you can see, cardiomyopathy can mean several things. The heart muscle can be thickened or not, and the heart itself can be mildly enlarged or very enlarged. The three main categories you should remember are dilated, restrictive, and hypertrophic cardiomyopathy. Of these, only hypertrophic involves significant heart muscle thickening.

Any heart chamber can be enlarged or hypertrophied, but the left ventricle is most commonly affected in clinical practice. If you remember that hypertrophy equals thickening equals larger deflections on the ECG, you'll see larger deflections over the precordial leads exactly where the thickening is located. You'll also see a right-axis deviation in RVH and left-axis deviation in LVH.

CHAPTER 7:
MYOCARDIAL ISCHEMIA AND INFARCTION

We've talked so much about rhythm disturbances in ECG tracings, we've almost forgotten why most ECGs are done in the emergency department. In the ED, people come to be seen all the time for chest pain, worried they are having a heart attack. Most of them aren't, thankfully, but they'll invariably get an ECG, regardless of how close their chest pain resembles that of an MI.

In this chapter, you'll learn the different syndromes linked to heart-related chest pain, and see how the ECG can be a valuable tool in helping the medical staff make a fairly clear distinction between noncardiac chest pain, ischemic heart disease, and a major myocardial infarction.

Ischemia versus Infarction

If given a choice over what kind of heart-related blood vessel disease one wanted, most would probably pick one involving ischemia rather than infarction. Ischemia just means the heart muscle is starved for oxygen. It sends out pain signals as an SOS to you and your healthcare provider, telling you to do something fast to avoid worsened conditions.

In some cases, you would only feel chest pain if you were exercising. When you slowed down or rested, the pain would go away. The reason for this is that coronary arterial blood flow is largely rate-dependent. As your heart rate increases, the time in diastole goes down. As you can imagine, very little blood can squeeze through the coronary arteries while the heart is itself squeezing in systole. Most blood gets to the muscles during diastole. As the time for diastole shrinks as the heart rate rises, less blood gets to the muscles.

Infarction, on the other hand, is basically "deadness of the heart." The blood flow has gone from okay to ischemia and, finally, to heart muscle death. Ischemia is reversible, but infarction is not. The degree to which you'll see infarction on the ECG depends on which vessel is blocked and how much dead tissue there is in the heart.

Options in the ED

If a person comes into the emergency department with chest pain and an ECG is done, you have a few options of conclusion to make:

- **Noncardiac chest pain is present.** The pain doesn't fit, and the ECG shows nothing suspicious. It may or may not be normal, but it will not show acute ischemic changes in the heart.
- **Stable angina is present.** The pain fits but has disappeared with rest or with oral nitroglycerin. This is a warning sign but nothing more. You do not need to rush out to do anything, and the ECG usually does not show any areas of ischemia.
- **Unstable angina is present.** The pain fits, doesn't go away easily, and the ECG may show specific or nonspecific changes indicating ischemia. You do not see a recent infarction on the ECG, but you still choose to keep this person and solve their blood vessel blockage issue.

- **NSTEMI is present.** The pain fits and doesn't go away easily (if at all). There is evidence of cardiac muscle death, but the ECG will specifically show that cell death in the heart does not go through the entire wall. NSTEMI means "non-ST-elevation MI."
- **STEMI is present.** The pain fits and doesn't go away easily (if at all). There is evidence of cardiac muscle death, and the ECG shows acute changes indicating the entire muscle wall is involved, from the epicardium through the endocardium.

NOTE: Unstable angina, NSTEMI, and STEMI are ALL acute coronary syndrome. You can breathe more easily if the chest pain is noncardiac or stable angina. All the rest need some type of urgent medical or surgical intervention.

When you see an NSTEMI, you can almost always assume that the heart muscle wall's inner lining/endocardium is damaged or dead, but that the outermost layer has been spared. Why would this be? Remember that the large coronary arteries encase the heart and travel in the epicardial layer. Branches from these larger arteries pierce the wall, so only the tiniest vessels reach the inner layers. If there is blockage of any coronary artery, the flow in these littlest arteries will be most affected.

Ischemia on ECG Tracings

Most ECG changes in ischemia are detected by looking at the ST segment or the T wave. The two things you'll see are 1) ST-segment depression greater than 1 mm, and 2) T wave inversion. Now that you have a mental picture of which leads most represent certain parts of the heart, you can guess where the ischemia is located. The more abnormal leads you see, the greater is the area of ischemia involved.

ST segment depression

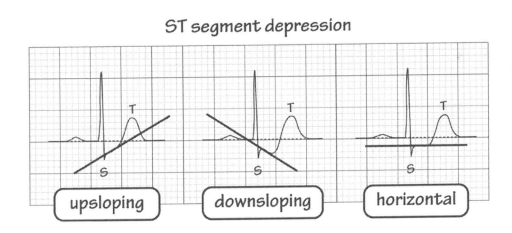

The best evidence of true ischemia will be ST-segment depression of more than 0.5 mm at the J point in at least two leads. Depression greater than this is a bad sign; depression greater than 2 mm in at least three leads is significant for an NSTEMI and not just ischemia. A third of these patients will be dead in a month. Upsloping ST depression is nonspecific and means less than horizontal or downsloping ST-segment depression. This next figure shows you where the J point is located.

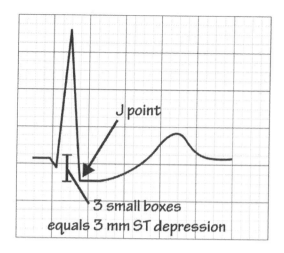

Don't forget that T wave inversion is another common sign of ischemia:

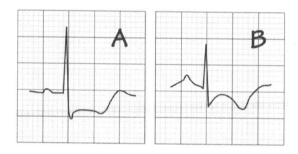

Telling the difference between myocardial ischemia (unstable angina) and an NSTEMI (infarction) often can't be done using the ECG alone. This is where cardiac enzymes come in. Heart muscle will only release cardiac enzymes from dead cells that have burst to release their contents (which include enzymes). If these are elevated, you've got an infarction; if not, you have unstable angina/ischemia.

Identifying a Myocardial Infarction

All you can say about myocardial ischemia is that it is either present or not present. It rarely leaves a trace, so if you don't catch it as it's happening, you may not know that it was present eight hours ago. Infarction is not that way. Not only can you usually identify it at the time it is happening, because there are dead myocardial muscle cells involved, but their absence will also often leave a trace, usually because a scar forms in the myocardium instead.

Certainly you need to get cardiac enzymes to prove cell death, but even elevations of those won't leave any kind of trace. So if a person presents to the emergency department saying they had chest pain three days ago, the enzymes may be normal; you need other options, like an echocardiogram, angiogram or ECG, to see if the chest pain event was a myocardial infarction.

There are a few things you can mostly count on in an infarction situation: 1) ST-segment elevation showing an injury is taking place; 2) Q waves on the ECG tracing, indicating necrosis has happened at some time in the past; and 3) T-wave inversion, showing both ischemia and the evolution of cell death in the heart. You must see these changes to expect your MI to be located in the patient's heart. They will be seen mainly in the leads facing the surface affected.

Because the ECG leads form an electrical grid of sorts, any major deflection in one lead will show an automatic reciprocal deflection in the opposite direction. Some reciprocal changes to look for are tall R waves opposite any leads where Q waves are seen. This is because R waves are the reciprocal deflection (mirror image) of any Q waves you see. Tall T waves also mirror T wave deflection elsewhere. This table gives you a rough idea of where to look:

SITE	FACING	RECIPROCAL
INFERIOR	II, III, aVF	I, aVL
HIGH LATERAL	I, aVL	II, III, aVF
ANTERIOR	V1, V2, V3, V4	NONE
POSTERIOR	NONE	V1, V2, V3, V4

The precordial leads can be beneficial. Think of them as wrapping around the sides and front of the heart, which is pretty much how you actually place them. You can hunt for changes in these, especially with anterior myocardial infarctions. This image should help you get the idea:

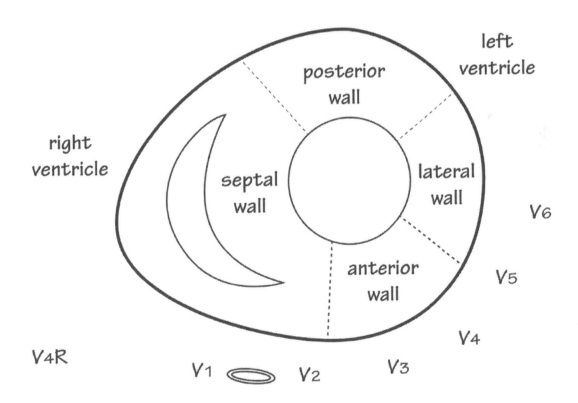

Since a myocardial infarction occurs or "evolves" over time, you should be able to use an ECG to some degree to help you tell if an MI is new, in the middle of its process, or long past the actual event. Here's what happens:

1. The T waves get tall and peaked—this happens so early that you may easily miss it, unless the person is being evaluated in the hospital when the MI begins.
2. The ST segment elevates—this indicates that injury has occurred to heart muscle cells. A STEMI is identified if the elevation is at least 1 mm and is confirmed in a neighboring lead that faces roughly the same direction. The larger the elevation of the ST segment, the more muscle is involved in that lead.

Q waves develop—these must be deep (25 percent or more of the total QRS height) and at least 0.03 seconds wide (three-fourths of a small box). These show up about 8 to 12 hours into the process or longer, and may never disappear. You can actually sum the entire thing up in one picture-story that looks a lot like this (hint: follow the numbers to see which changes occur and when you see them):

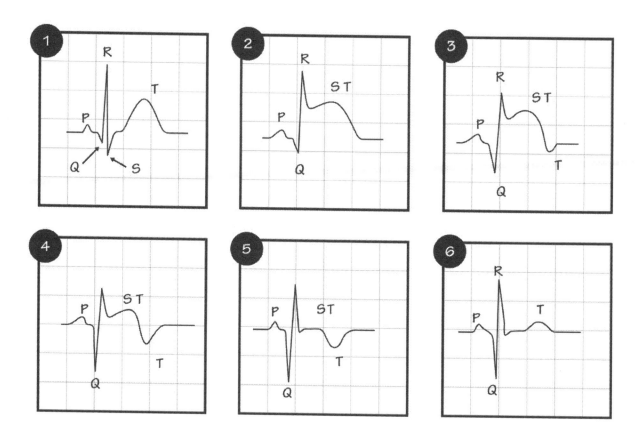

You can memorize what each type of MI looks like on an ECG, but that's actually a waste of your time. It is far better to remember the image of the leads superimposed on the heart. Where you see evidence of infarction on any lead, confirm its presence with any neighboring lead, or look for mirror-image changes in an opposite lead. This will give you your answer.

This image also helps a lot:

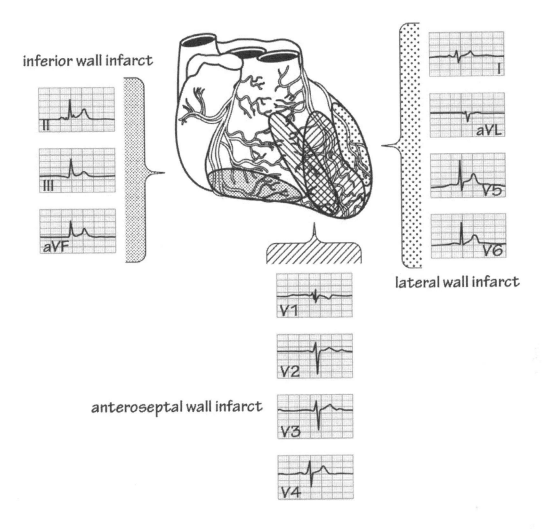

inferior wall infarct

lateral wall infarct

anteroseptal wall infarct

If you are a budding cardiologist and want to know which vessel to expect your occlusion, you need only track it with this handy table:

Description	ECG leads with changes	Artery occluded
Inferior	II, III, aVF	RCA
Anteroapical	V3 and V4	Distal LAD
Anteroseptal	V1 and V2	LAD
Anterolateral	I, aVL, V5 and V6	Circumflex artery
Extensive anterior	I, aVL, V2-V6	Proximal LCA
True posterior	Tall R in V1	RCA
True posterior	Tall R in V1	RCA

So far, we've been covering the STEMI or transmural MI. It travels all the way to affect the entire thickness of heart muscle in a given area. In an NSTEMI, only the heart wall's innermost parts are affected, so what you'll see is very different. Let's compare a STEMI and an NSTEMI on an ECG so you can see the obvious difference between the two types.

NSTEMI versus STEMI

Since you were allowed to pick whether you wanted to have ischemia or infarction, it's only fair to let you also choose between having a STEMI or an NSTEMI. Hopefully, you've decided on an NSTEMI because this is less dangerous than a STEMI. The main reason for this is that a STEMI is transmural (through the wall). The chances of complications of an MI, such as a wall rupture, aneurysm, heart failure or arrhythmia, are much greater if the entire heart muscle wall is affected, compared to just a part of it.

TRICK QUESTION: If the ECG is normal, does that mean there is no MI? Of course not. A normal ECG can be seen in any MI, especially an NSTEMI. You may have missed the changes, or you will see them later. It's hard to make this kind of diagnosis without serial (over time) enzymes and ECGs. Don't get burned by thinking a normal one means the patient is set to go!

In an NSTEMI, the ECG will have its own set of changes, but they are far less obvious. You can essentially see anything on an NSTEMI. You would see if a person simply had ischemia: T wave inversion and ST-segment depression in the leads facing or overlying the infarcted area. Of course, the main difference is that the cardiac enzymes will be elevated in a true NSTEMI, while you won't see enzyme elevation in unstable angina/ischemia. You will also never see Q waves in an NSTEMI.

This image explains why you will see ST-segment depression in an NSTEMI (partial wall thickness injury) and ST-segment elevation in a STEMI. The arrows show where the electricity travels in each case. If the arrows travel toward the lead, the ST segment will be elevated. If the arrows travel in the opposite direction, the deflection will be below the line (ST-segment depression).

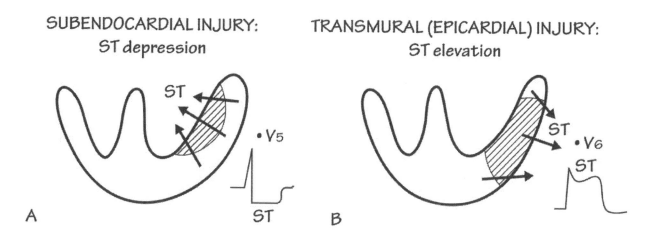

To Sum Things Up

Injury to heart muscle spans a wide range, from simple transient lack of circulation during exercise to muscle cell death that spans the entirety of the cardiac muscle wall. The ECG will not always be able to tell you for certain that an MI has occurred (it may look normal), but if you combine repeated/serial ECGs and serial enzymes in the workup of chest pain, you will be well on your way to determining whether or not a heart attack/MI is occurring or has happened.

CHAPTER 8:
ELECTROLYTES AND DRUG EFFECTS

You might think the only real reason to perform an ECG is because of some heart-related symptoms, such as chest pains, syncope, or palpitations. In actuality, you will do many more ECGs for things like electrolyte disturbances and drug overdoses or toxicities than you might think. Because electrolytes are a natural part of the electrochemistry of the heart muscle cells, abnormalities in these may adversely affect the heart.

The two major electrolytes involved in heart muscle contractility are potassium and calcium. Drugs will also affect the heart. There are also several drugs that are notorious for affecting the heart, including digoxin, beta-blockers, and calcium channel blockers, each of which acts on the heart in some way under normal circumstances. One other you will encounter is the class of drugs called tricyclic antidepressants. These are not cardiac drugs, but can have profound actions on the heart if taken as an overdose.

Hyperkalemia

Probably the most dangerous electrolyte disturbance you'll encounter is hyperkalemia. When you know the patient has hyperkalemia, the ECG is confirmatory; other times, the ECG will demonstrate something suspicious enough to alert providers that hyperkalemia is likely present.

The main risk of hyperkalemia is the development of sudden arrhythmia, leading to ventricular tachycardia or sudden cardiac death from ventricular fibrillation. Fortunately, there are specific findings you'll see on an ECG that can clue you in that this electrolyte disturbance is present.

A normal potassium level is between 3.5 and 5.2 mEq/liter. When you see ECG changes, they will evolve from normal to very severe as the potassium progresses. This is great because you can predict the potassium level by what you see on the ECG. These are the stepwise changes you should be able to recognize:

1. When the potassium is between 5.5 and 6.5 mEq/l, the T waves will be peaked with a narrow base, particularly if you look in the precordial leads. You might also see a short QT interval and some ST segment depression. Peaked T waves look like this:

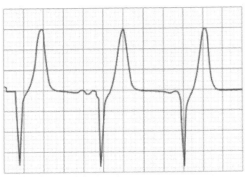

2. When the potassium is between 6.5 and 8.0 mEq/l, you will start to see other changes. These include prolonged PR intervals, low amplitude P waves, widened QRS complex, and an amplified R wave on the QRS complex. You will see these changes as shown:

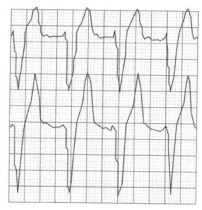

3. These changes worsen over time, so you will see what's called a "sine wave pattern." This is almost always fatal to the patient.

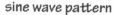

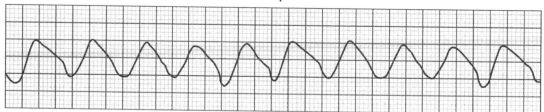

In a pinch (i.e. when you are trying desperately to save someone from what will probably quickly be fatal), giving potassium should NOT be your first choice. Instead, give IV calcium, which protects the heart for a brief period of time. Ultimately, things like insulin, Lasix, albuterol, and bicarbonate will help pull potassium from inside the cells to outside (which will also help). Finally, giving IV potassium will make the greatest long-term difference in outcomes.

ONE EXCEPTION: *Do not give IV calcium if the patient has high potassium levels because of digoxin toxicity. You will probably kill the patient if you do this.*

Hypokalemia

Hypokalemia is not good for the heart either, but generally isn't as severe as hyperkalemia. You will usually see ECG changes if the potassium is below 3.0 mEq/l. Look for the presence of a U wave with a lesser deflection than in the T wave. The T wave will also be flatter, and the ST segment can look like ischemia with ST-segment depression. Look for these typical findings:

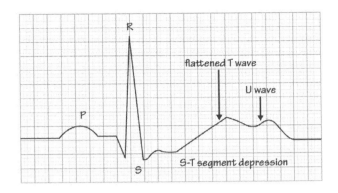

If the potassium level is below 2.5 mEq/l, you might see an inverted T wave as well. The main treatment for these ECG findings is to replace the lost potassium.

Hypercalcemia

Hypercalcemia (high calcium levels) can also be seen on an ECG. You might expect to encounter a variety of changes that will take a practiced eye to see:

- Shortened QT interval
- Osborne waves
- Shortened ST segment

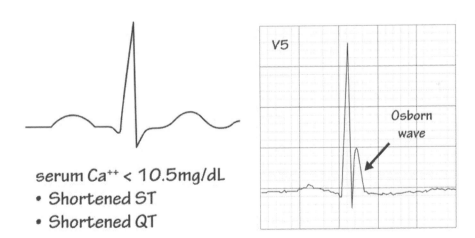

Just remember that the length of everything from the start of the Q wave to the end of the T wave gets shorter.

Hypocalcemia

The findings you'll see with hypocalcemia (low calcium levels) is essentially the opposite of what you'll see when the calcium level is too high. Notably, look for a long QT interval and a prolonged ST segment. Everything in hypercalcemia is compressed, while everything in hypocalcemia is stretched out. It might look like this:

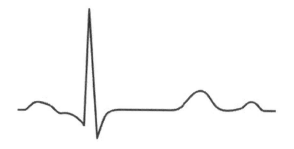

serum Ca++ < 8.5mg/dL
- Lengthened ST
- Lengthened QT
- May cause Torsades de pointes

A long QT situation is a bit vague, because there are other causes of a long QT (including genetic conditions). If you see this, you'll have a wider workup to consider. These findings can also lead to Torsades de Pointes.

Drug effects on ECG Tracings

Digoxin isn't used much for heart failure anymore, mostly because it is too easy to become toxic. The most common sign of high levels and toxicity from digoxin is some type of ECG change. In reality, many ECG changes might be seen, but the most common one is a downslope of the ST segment in what's called the "reverse check sign," because it looks like a backward checkmark. It looks like this:

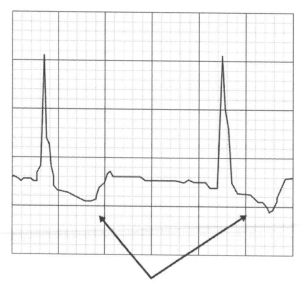

"reverse check" or "reverse tick"
sign from digoxin effect

Many different rhythm disturbances can come from being toxic from digoxin, but the two you won't see are atrial flutter and atrial fibrillation (with rapid rates). One common one is atrial tachycardia with 2:1 conduction of the P waves. You may also see certain types of ventricular tachycardia or atrial fibrillation, along with a slow ventricular response.

Beta-Blockers and Calcium-Channel Blockers

Beta-blockers (like atenolol, propranolol and sotalol) and certain cardio-selective calcium-channel blockers (like diltiazem and verapamil) will show problems if used at toxic levels. You should see some nonspecific findings on the ECG indicating that there are toxic concentrations of some of these drug classes, including:

- Junctional bradycardia
- Sinus bradycardia
- AV block (first through third degree)

Note that each of these involves some type of bradycardia or slow heart rate. If you see a long PR interval and nothing else, this will be an early sign of possible toxicity.

Two beta-blockers stand out as having unique changes in an ECG if there is toxicity of any kind. Propranolol often causes coma, seizures or hypotension when a person is toxic. This is because the fast sodium channels in the heart and brain are affected at the same time. In the heart, the effect is an ECG with a widening of the QRS complex and an R' wave seen in aVR. If not managed, the CNS effects plus ventricular arrhythmias will be seen.

Sotalol blocks the potassium channels in the heart, which prolongs the QT interval. Anytime you see QT prolongation, you need to think that Torsades de Pointes might be a complication of this issue.

Tricyclic Antidepressants and Others

Tricyclic antidepressants fall into the class of sodium channel blockers. A more common drug like this can be toxic to the heart after an overdose. Other sodium-channel blockers include:

- Quinidine or procainamide (type Ia antiarrhythmic drugs)
- Flecainide (and other types Ic antiarrhythmic drugs)
- Local anesthetics (like bupivacaine)
- Hydroxychloroquine or chloroquine (antimalarials)
- Carbamazepine
- Quinine

These drugs all do different things but each have the effect of blocking sodium channels, so the effect on the heart will be similar (when toxic). An ECG can be very helpful in making a diagnosis of a sodium-channel blocker toxicity situation. You might notice any one of these things:

- Interventricular conduction delay with a prolonged QRS interval
- Right axis deviation with a high R-to-S ratio in aVR
- R' wave seen in aVR

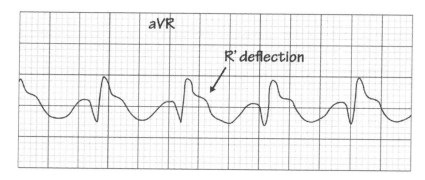

- Sinus tachycardia in tricyclic overdoses (because of blockage of some parasympathetic receptors in the body)

The end result is that two of the major side effects are seizures and ventricular arrhythmias, which can be lethal if the overdose is significant enough. Tricyclic antidepressants also inhibit the potassium channels, which accounts for a prolongation of the QT interval. The myocardial muscle strength is depressed overall, so that you will see hypotension/shock as well.

If the QRS is longer than 100 ms in a tricyclic antidepressant overdose setting, the risk of seizures is high. If the QRS is greater than 160 ms, the risk of VTach or other dangerous ventricular arrhythmias will be an additional factor. This is why an ECG is essential in an overdose situation. When the patient is unconscious, he or she will not be able to tell you what they've taken, and it could well be a tricyclic antidepressant overdose (or a combination of drugs that includes that one).

To Sum Things Up

Most people don't think much past the heart when looking at an ECG. They forget that the heart muscle operates because of molecular, biological, and biochemical pathways, and that it isn't just a structural organ. For this reason, you need to think about the effects of drugs and electrolytes on the heart muscle.

In fact, there are drugs and electrolyte disturbances that will kill a person at any age, even if the heart itself is normal. Potassium and calcium abnormalities are major culprits, while drugs acting on the electrolyte channels in the heart muscle cells also have a major impact on how the electrical pathways of the heart are supposed to work.

Made in the USA
Columbia, SC
28 January 2022

54943891R00087